DATE			

Critical Issues in Health and Medicine

Edited by Rima D. Apple, University of Wisconsin–Madison,
and Janet Golden, Rutgers University, Camden

Growing criticism of the U.S. health care system is coming from consumers,
politicians, the media, activists, and healthcare professionals. Critical Issues in
Health and Medicine is a collection of books that explores these contemporary
dilemmas from a variety of perspectives, among them political, legal, historical,
sociological, and comparative, and with attention to crucial dimensions such as
race, gender, ethnicity, sexuality, and culture.

For a list of titles in the series, see the last page of the book.

The Morning After

A History of Emergency Contraception in the United States

Heather Munro Prescott

Rutgers University Press

New Brunswick, New Jersey, and London

Library of Congress Cataloging-in-Publication Data

Prescott, Heather Munro.

The morning after : a history of emergency contraception in the United States /
Heather Munro Prescott.

p.   cm.   — (Critical issues in health and medicine)
Includes bibliographical references and index.

ISBN 978–0–8135–5162–3 (hardcover : alk. paper) —
ISBN 978–0–8135–5163–0 (pbk. : alk. paper)
1. Emergency contraceptives—United States—History. 2. Birth control—United States.
I. Title.
RG137.5.P74 2011
618.1'825—dc22

2011004711

A British Cataloging-in-Publication record for this book is available from the British Library.

Visit our Web site: http://rutgerspress.rutgers.edu

Manufactured in the United States of America

Typesetting: BookType

For my family

Contents

Acknowledgments

The idea for this book originated from a paper I presented at the annual meeting of the Society for the History of Technology held in Amsterdam in 2004. I thank Sharra Vostral for thinking of me when she was looking for a last-minute replacement for a panelist who had to drop out unexpectedly. I thought that this project would end with the conference paper and perhaps an article in the society's journal, but session commenter Andre Tone suggested that this subject deserved a book-length treatment. Series editors Rima Apple and Janet Golden encouraged me to submit this manuscript to the Rutgers University Press series Critical Issues in Health and Medicine. I am grateful to the Press's director, Marlie Wasserman, and editors Doreen Valentine and Peter Mickulas for guiding this project from submission to final product.

Internal and external research funding was essential to the completion of this book. Faculty Research Grants from the Connecticut State University–American Association of University Professors funded the extensive travel to archives needed to complete research for this project. National Institutes of Health Publication Grant LM 009242–01A2, sponsored by the Office of Research on Women's Health, reduced my teaching load so that I could dedicate half of my time to writing and revision. I am thankful to Mimi Kaplan and Dean Kleinert from my university's Grants and Funded Research Office and NIH Program officer Hua-Chuan Sim for helping me submit successful grant proposals.

There are numerous archivists and librarians who have helped me with the research on this project. At Central Connecticut State University, I am especially indebted to the tireless efforts of interlibrary loan librarian Kimberly Farrington and her staff for their speed and efficiency in handling my voluminous requests. At the American College of Obstetricians and Gynecologists, resource center director Mary Hyde, history librarian and archivist Debra Scarborough, and reference librarian Pamela Van Hine provided invaluable assistance in finding resources not only from ACOG but from individual reproductive health care professionals and feminist health organizations. Stephen Greenberg and Elizabeth Fee at the National Library of Medicine, National Institutes of Health, also deserve thanks for their help and support. Historians Suzanne White Junod and John Swann from the Food and Drug Administration History Office shared their expert knowledge and helped me locate materials on the agency's role in promoting and regulating emergency contraception. I am also grateful to Susan Boone, reference librarian at the Sophia Smith Collection at Smith College, and Ellen M. Shea, head of reference at the Arthur and Elizabeth Schlesinger Library on the History of Women in America at Radcliffe Institute for Advanced Study, for helping me navigate the various collections on women and reproductive rights housed in those libraries. I would like to acknowledge Malgosia Myc from the Bentley Historical Library at the University of Michigan for locating the artist Germaine Keller, who created the image from the feminist periodical *her-self* used in chapter 3. I thank Ms. Keller for granting permission to use this image.

Various reproductive health care professionals and women's health activists have offered me insight and advice into the development of their field. Many of these individuals are named throughout the text and include Amy Allina, Marie Bass, Kelly Blanchard, Sharon Camp, Renee Chelian, Kelly Cleland, Belita Cowan, Margaret Johnson, Claire Keyes, Kirsten Moore, Judy Norsigian, Megan Peterson, James Trussell, Elizabeth Westley, and the late Barbara Seaman. Special thanks go to Drs. Ernest Kohorn and Philip Sarrell, who helped flesh out the story of early work on the "morning-after pill" at Yale–New Haven Hospital. I have also benefited greatly from the expert knowledge and extensive collection of papers of Dr. Takey Crist. Canadian obstetrician/gynecologist Al Yuzpe shared with me his memories of developing the emergency contraceptive regimen that bears his name. I am extremely grateful to Lisa Wynn for sharing her work-in-progress and tacit knowledge about the various individuals and organizations that work on emergency contraception in the United States. Morganne Rosenhaus from the Reproductive Health Technologies Project and Jane Gauthier and Jenny Lacombe from the Canadian Federation for Sexual Health were a great help in obtaining images for this book.

Many thanks go to various friends and colleagues who have read and commented on this work as it progressed from conference papers to the final manuscript. In addition to the series editors and outside reviewer Rebecca Kluchin, these include Andrea Tone, Nelly Oudshoorn, Elizabeth Siegel Watkins, Johann Schoen, Wendy Kline, Leslie Reagan, Naomi Rogers, Judith Houck, and Ellen More. Most of all, I would like to thank my husband, Wayne, and the rest of my family for their love and support during the years it took to complete this project.

Abbreviations

AMA	American Medical Association
AMI	Advocates for Medical Information
BWHBC	Boston Women's Health Book Collective
CARASA	Committee for Abortion Rights and Against Sterilization Abuse
CDER	Center for Drug Evaluation and Research, Food and Drug Administration
CMRW	Coalition for Medical Rights of Women
CRLP	Center for Reproductive Law and Policy
CRR	Center for Reproductive Rights
DES	diethylstilbestrol
FDA	Food and Drug Administration
KFF	Kaiser Family Foundation
MAPC	Morning-After Pill Conspiracy
NICHHD	National Institute for Child Health and Human Development
NOW	National Organization for Women
NWHN	National Women's Health Network
PATH	Program for Appropriate Technology in Health
PIWH	Pacific Institute for Women's Health
RHTP	Reproductive Health Technologies Project
WFEB	Worcester Foundation for Experimental Biology

The Morning After

Introduction

I first heard about emergency contraception during the 1990s, when a cluster of stories about a "back-up" method of birth control appeared in medical journals, popular magazines, and televised news reports, including a program on the popular music channel MTV. Although I was an assistant professor working on the history of adolescent health issues, and involved in reproductive rights activism on campus and in the community, I had not heard of emergency contraception before. Like others, I assumed that this was a relatively new contraceptive technology. As I was researching my last book on the history of college health, I discovered that this media campaign was the culmination of decades of efforts by reproductive health professionals and women's health activists to make emergency contraception widely available in the United States.

This book is the first to describe the history of emergency contraception from its beginnings in the 1960s. Other historical accounts of this technology focus on the very recent past and present a story of uniform progress from "the nation's best kept secret" to a dedicated product found on most pharmacy shelves.[1] In these histories, there are clearly delineated opposing positions: on one side are those who support the technology as an uncomplicated scientific solution to the problem of unwanted pregnancy; on the other are religious conservatives who seek to ban the technology because they erroneously equate it with abortion.

Yet there is a much longer history of emergency contraception, one that is intertwined with the larger history of contraceptive research and reproductive politics in the United States. Like the history of birth control more generally, it is a complex story that includes reproductive scientists, population control groups, healthcare providers, feminist health activists, pharmaceutical companies, regulatory agencies, and legislators. These individuals and organizations have often held conflicting opinions and goals. Moreover, their perspectives have not remained constant but have changed significantly over the last half-century. Even the technology of emergency contraception has evolved since it was first discovered in the mid 1960s. Today, the most common method of emergency contraception used in the United States is the product Plan B and its generic equivalents, which can be used up to seventy-two hours after unprotected sex. These products are composed of the synthetic progesterone levonorgestral. In 2010, the FDA approved the emergency contraceptive ellaOne, containing the compound ulipristal acetate, which extends the period of effectiveness to five days. Certain brands of regular oral contraceptive pills, containing both progesterone and estrogen, can also be used for emergency contraception. The Copper-T intraruterine device (IUD), more typically used for regular birth control, can prevent pregnancy if inserted within five days of unprotected sex.[2]

In addition, the words used to describe what is now called emergency contraception have changed over time, and this book reflects these shifts in terminology. The scientists who first discovered this technology used the term "postcoital contraception" to indicate that this method was to be used after intercourse. The popular press soon coined the term "morning-after pill" to describe this contraceptive method. Although this colloquialism was inaccurate, it remained in popular use until the early 1990s. Since then, advocates have used the term "emergency contraception" to both correct misperceptions about the time frame for taking the drug as well as emphasize that this should not be used as an ongoing method of birth control.

In the past, various other chemical compounds have been used as emergency contraceptives. The scientists who developed these compounds did not purposely set out to invent this birth control method. Rather, this technology grew out of scientific research on female hormones more generally. While some of this research was devoted to finding an effective oral contraceptive, scientists were just as interested in finding treatments for infertility and the unpleasant aspects of menopause. In addition, scientists and the population groups who funded them were not necessarily invested in the reproductive rights of American women, even though they received financial and political support from the prominent birth control advocates Margaret Sanger and Katherine McCormack. One of the developers of the Pill, John Rock, for example, supported birth control because it would improve marital happiness, not because it would empower women. Moreover, concerns about the social problems that emerged from overpopulation in both the United States and the developing world frequently overshadowed the issue of female autonomy in making reproductive choices.[3] This tension between a disease model intended to "cure" unwanted pregnancy and a reproductive rights framework aimed at increasing women's birth control choices runs throughout the history of emergency contraception in the United States.

The earliest substances used for postcoital contraception were synthetic estrogens, first developed in the 1930s for hormone replacement therapy. Although scientists in the 1950s and 1960s demonstrated the effectiveness of several synthetic estrogens, the nonsteroidal estrogen diethylstilbestrol (DES) became the method of choice because it was more potent and less expensive to manufacture than other synthetic estrogens. It also could be taken orally rather than through intramuscular injection.[4] DES was also approved to treat women with various pregnancy complications, including toxemia and gestational diabetes, as well as reduce the likelihood of miscarriage. During the early 1970s, oncologists discovered that DES caused a rare form of malignant vaginal cancer in the daughters of women who had taken the drug during pregnancy. Although there was no evidence that using DES as an emergency contraceptive could cause cancer, all applications of the drug came under scrutiny as part of a larger feminist critique of how the medical profession mistreated women.[5]

This feminist critique shaped not only healthcare policy, but also the historiography of women's healthcare. Feminist scholars showed that medical science both past and present was not objective or neutral, but rather was shaped by sexist attitudes about women and their proper place in society.[6] More recently, historians of women's healthcare history, while recognizing the value of this groundbreaking work, have also challenged some of the assumptions of early feminist scholarship. Instead, they have traced a more nuanced history of the relationship between women and the medical profession. In particular, this more recent work has tried to capture the experience of female patients. These historians show that rather than being passive victims, women had an active role in shaping the kind of care they received. In the case of birth control, historians have restored historical agency to women who were among the first to use the contraceptive pill and other reproductive technologies.[7]

My analysis also draws on points made by Adele Clarke and Theresa Montini's work on RU 486 (mifepristone). As Clarke and Montini argue, contraceptives are examples of "contested technologies" which are "constructed within as well as disseminated through extant, contentious arenas composed of heterogeneous actors committed to action on the core issue." Clarke and Montini offer an "arena analysis" of the "various actors, including scientists, pharmaceutical companies, medical groups, antiabortion groups, women's health movement groups, and others who have produced situated knowledges" of RU 486.[8] Likewise, this book will explore the multiple constituencies involved in the development and marketing of emergency contraceptives since the 1960s. Because various forms of emergency contraception have existed since the 1960s, this technology has a significantly longer history than does mifepristone. Therefore, it is possible to trace not only the "heterogeneous constructions" of this technology by various actors, but also how the attitudes of some key participants involved in this story have evolved over time.

The book is organized chronologically to demonstrate how the story of emergency contraception fits within the larger history of birth control politics and drug regulation in the United States. Chapter 1 examines how emergency contraception appeared at a critical moment in the history of contraceptive research and development in the 1960s. Work of reproductive scientists and population experts during this era reflected what Johanna Schoen calls the "complex set of factors that motivated health and welfare professionals' involvement in the delivery of birth control" to indigent populations in the United States. On the one hand, many of these professionals were "genuinely concerned with maternal and child health and hoped to improve women's access to health and contraceptive services." On the other hand, they also argued, "The distribution of contraceptives among the poor would save taxpayers money by controlling state expenses for social services."[9] Although by the 1960s, some health professionals were beginning the express the view that even the poor had a right to reproductive autonomy, there was also a persistent belief that poor, uneducated women were unreliable contraceptors. Consequently, these professionals tended to favor technologies, such as the IUD, that did not require client cooperation and could be solely under the control of physicians rather than patients. The so-called morning-after pill was one of the methods developed to address the "disease" of unwanted pregnancy.

Chapter 2 examines how this disease-based approach continued to shape medical and popular discourse about the morning-after pill as this birth control method became part of the reproductive health options offered to women at the nation's colleges and universities. This chapter focuses on the work of Yale researchers John McLean Morris and Gertrude van Wagenen, who tested postcoital DES on patients at Yale–New Haven Hospital and the student health service at Yale University. I argue that the development and dissemination of the morning-after pill responded in part to social anxieties about the impact of the era's "sexual revolution" on the behavior of young women. At the same time, some birth control professionals realized that sexual violence and social inequality were contributing factors to the "disease" of unwanted pregnancy.

Chapter 3 explores the controversy surrounding the use of DES as a postcoital contraceptive and sets this debate within the larger context of feminist critiques of hormonal contraception. It focuses on the work of Advocates for Medical Information (AMI), forerunner of the National Women's Health Network (NWHN). This group was part of a larger effort by health feminists to expose various abuses of women at the hands of the medical profession. Feminist health activists called attention to serious ethical lapses in the treatment of human subjects. They argued that young women served as "guinea pigs" for this new drug while doctors failed to observe professional standards of informed consent. They claimed that giving DES as a postcoital contraceptive to young women who had already been exposed to the drug in utero was unethical and heightened their risk of developing cancer. At the heart of this critique was a challenge to the disease-based approach to birth control promoted by most reproductive health professionals.

Chapter 4 examines the impact of these feminist critiques on further developments in contraceptive research and development. Concerns about the dangers of DES raised by feminist health activists led researchers to search for new drugs that could be used as postcoital contraceptives. Yet, researchers retained the same disease model that had driven the development of the first morning-after pill. This chapter will also examine how patient demand for this reproductive technology persisted even as protests from women's health activists escalated. This chapter will show how these women consumers made healthcare choices within a complex medical, political, and regulatory environment.

Chapter 5 explores the shifting attitudes of feminist health activists toward emergency contraception. It focuses on the changing position of the National Women's Health Network (NWHN), at first a vehement critic of hormonal contraceptive methods. The increasingly conservative political climate regarding birth control and abortion prompted the organization to reevaluate its position and join broader efforts to develop a dedicated product for what activists now called emergency contraception. This chapter will show how emergency contraception became an issue that bridged gaps between radical feminist organizations such as NWHN and politically moderate women's groups and reproductive health professionals.

Chapter 6 looks at how this collaboration of former adversaries played a central role in increasing awareness of emergency contraception through a nationwide media campaign and in convincing the FDA to approve dedicated products packaged exclusively for this purpose. This chapter looks at the development of the emergency contraceptive products Preven and Plan B and shows how these products represented innovative approaches to drug production and marketing in the United States.

Chapter 7 looks at recent efforts to make emergency contraception available over the counter. It demonstrates how this was part of a larger trend toward "do-it-yourself" medicine and the growing availability of over-the-counter (OTC) drugs and home testing kits. This chapter places the story of OTC Plan B within a longer history of women's activism on behalf of consumer protection and reproductive rights. This activism not only helped make emergency contraception available without a prescription, but also led many reproductive health professionals to reject the disease-based approach to contraceptive innovation in favor of one that emphasized women's rights to reproductive choice. Experts who supported the OTC switch often used the same language as feminist health activists from the 1970s, arguing that women should be freed from the "paternalistic" doctor-patient relationship embodied in the prescription.

This book is intended to contribute to recent scholarship on how women have used experience of the physical body as a source of knowledge production and feminist practice regarding women's health issues.[10] Like these works, I use the history of emergency contraception to illuminate key themes in the politics of women's health since the 1960s. I argue that recent developments in the history of emergency contraception represent a major rapprochement between mainstream population control groups, representatives from the pharmaceutical industry, and members of feminist women's health advocacy groups. I show how these diverse groups created a middle ground between an older liberal feminist position that tended to support technological innovations such as hormonal contraception and a more radical feminist position that criticized the abuse of female human subjects by the medical profession but was otherwise in favor of reproductive rights. This story provides important lessons for those who hope to expand women's contraceptive options in the future.

Chapter 1

A Second Revolution in Birth Control

In a 1966 article in the *New York Times* magazine, abortion activist and investigative reporter Lawrence Lader celebrated the revolutionary accomplishments of the three "fathers" of the contraceptive pill: Dr. Gregory Pincus, research director of the Worcester Foundation for Experimental Biology (WFEB) in Shrewsbury, Massachusetts; WFEB senior research scientist Min Chueh Chang; and obstetrician-gynecologist John Rock, head of the Rock Reproductive Clinic in Brookline, Massachusetts. The article also announced studies by Pincus and Chang on a new development that could "herald a second revolution in birth control." This new "morning-after pill" could prevent conception after ovulation by accelerating the egg's progress through the reproductive tract and reducing the chances of fertilization. In addition to providing a back-up method of birth control, the new pill offered several advantages over existing oral contraceptives. Because it only had to be taken once, within a few days of intercourse, instead of every day, the new pill was less expensive. Therefore, it was a boon for women who lacked health insurance and were unable to afford the cost of regular birth control pills.[1]

The notion that the development of the Pill grew from the work of a small group of medical researchers is really a historical myth generated in part by memoirs written by these scientists and their collaborators.[2] These accounts frequently downplay the crucial role of reproductive rights pioneer Margaret Sanger, who fought for women's access to reliable contraception for decades, and Katherine McCormick, who provided generous funding to Pincus, Chang, and Rock at a time when no governmental agency and few private organizations were willing to support such controversial research.[3] Furthermore, the discovery of the Pill did not emerge sui generis: rather, it relied on earlier work in reproductive endocrinology and steroid chemistry conducted in the late nineteenth and early twentieth centuries that provided the foundation for the development of the first hormonal contraceptives. Finally, scientists in this field were not initially interested in finding methods of preventing pregnancy: rather, they were searching for the causes of infertility and other female reproductive disorders.

Nevertheless, by all accounts, the development of both the original oral contraceptive pill and the morning-after pill were revolutionary. These innovations provided women with birth control that was nearly 100 percent effective if used perfectly.[4] Yet the story of the morning-after pill is more than an interesting footnote to the larger history of the Pill. Although the popularity of this birth control method exceeded the wildest dreams of both Sanger and the scientists who developed this technology, by the mid-1960s the limitations of oral contraceptives were already becoming apparent. Scattered reports of women who had died or became seriously ill while on the Pill began to appear in the medical literature within a few years of the drug's approval in 1960.[5]

At the same time, physicians and scientists became concerned about the issue of noncompliance—that is, women who failed to use oral contraceptives optimally. Soon after the approval of the Pill, the first long-acting, reversible method of contraception, the intrauterine device (IUD) was reintroduced to the American market. Population experts claimed that the IUD was an ideal birth control method for low-income, poorly educated women whom they believed were less capable of remembering to take a daily pill.[6] The IUD was also considered an ideal method for unmarried teenagers because a young woman did not have to worry about a parent finding a package of oral contraceptives. Some physicians argued that even highly educated, married women were apt to forget to take their pills if they were too busy or they were "conflicted" about preventing pregnancy. In 1962, engineer David Wagner patented a package called the Dialpak dispenser to help women remember to take their pills daily.[7] These developments reflected the mixture of benevolence and paternalism that motivated birth control research in the United States. On the one hand, many of these professionals hoped to improve maternal and child health by removing legal and logistical barriers to women's access to health and contraceptive services. On the other hand, they also believed that limiting reproduction among the poor would provide a scientific solution to poverty and its attendant health problems.[8]

One of the new methods developed to deal with user error was the so-called morning-after pill.

From Infertility to Antifertility

The work of British physiologists A. S. Parkes and C. W. Bellerby at University College, London, in the 1920s laid the foundation for research that would lead to the development of the first postcoital methods of contraception. During a normal menstrual or estrus cycle, the follicle surrounding a mature egg forms a corpus luteum that secretes estrogen and progesterone. These two hormones are responsible for the thickening of the uterine lining and its maintenance during pregnancy. If the mature egg is not fertilized, it is expelled during menstruation, and the corpus luteum normally decays and is absorbed by the body. Parkes and Bellerby found that injection of high doses of the estrogen compound estradiol into rats and mice destroyed the corpus luteum and caused the rapid reappearance of the estrus cycle.[9]

Gregory Pincus duplicated these studies in both mice and rabbits during the mid-1930s. He and his collaborator H. O. Burdick discovered that injection of estradiol could not only interrupt pregnancy but also prevent it if administered within a few days of copulation.[10]

In 1938, Parkes, E. C. Dodds, and R. L. Noble demonstrated that the newly discovered synthetic estrogen compounds ethinyl estradiol and diethylstilbestrol (DES) could also be used as postcoital contraceptives. These compounds also could be administered by mouth rather than by injection, thereby making them more practical for use in humans. Parkes and his colleagues speculated that because the menstrual cycle in primates appeared to be similar to that of lower animals, their findings should also be applicable to women. However, the large amount of estrogen secreted during human pregnancy suggested that the period after intercourse during which estrogen treatment might be effective would be much shorter in humans than in rabbits.[11]

Although the implications of this research for developing contraceptives were clear, these scientists were mainly interested in using these findings for treatment of various reproductive disorders in animals and humans. Pincus's research on mammalian eggs was initially aimed at solving fertility problems in the field of animal husbandry. Even then, his work could not escape controversy. After discovering that estrogen compounds affected egg transport in rabbits, Pincus sought other ways to improve mammalian reproduction. Inspired by similar work on amphibian eggs, Pincus experimented with various compounds that could cause rabbit eggs to divide even in the absence of sperm. When word of Pincus's work became public, religious authorities roundly condemned it for violating the will of God. *Time* magazine coined the word "pincogenic" to describe these "unnatural" births. When Pincus suggested that this technique could be replicated in humans, the *New York Times* declared that a "brave new world" of "test tube babies" was on the horizon. The negative publicity following these experiments, which other researchers were unable to duplicate, combined with the rampant anti-Semitism of the era, led to the termination of Pincus's appointment at Harvard.[12]

Pincus's former Harvard classmate Hudson Hoagland, who was chair of the biology department at Clark University, learned of Pincus's predicament and offered him a position as visiting professor of experimental biology. Because the university had no funds for visiting appointments, Pincus's position was funded by a grant from the pharmaceutical company G. D. Searle to study the affects of anticonvulsants in test animals. Hoagland and Pincus eventually tired of the academic politics at Clark and in 1944 founded the private Worcester Foundation for Experimental Biology (WFEB). The WFEB quickly earned a reputation as a leader in steroid research by performing critical studies of the influence of hormones in cancer, arthritis, schizophrenia, and other mental illnesses. Within a few years a quarter of the foundation's annual budget was being provided by Searle pharmaceuticals. Officials at Searle hoped the foundation would help the company corner the market on the mass production of cortisone, a highly effective steroid treatment for arthritis.[13]

Pincus also continued his research on factors affecting mammalian fertility and in 1945 accepted an application from Chang to join the research team at the WFEB. Chang was especially interested in furthering Pincus's work on in-vitro fertilization and soon became an authority on substances that could enhance the fertilizing capabilities of mammalian sperm. Chang also did key studies on factors affecting sperm motility and capacitation (the ability of sperm to fertilize an egg) in the female reproductive tract. Like Pincus, while Chang's main interest was in treating infertility, his work also had implications for contraceptive research since the same principles could be used to inhibit rather than improve the chances of fertilization.[14]

John Rock also began his career treating cases of infertility in women at the Free Hospital for Women in Brookline during the 1930s. His work became even more critical as the stigma surrounding childlessness intensified during the Baby Boom that followed the Second World War.[15] Like Pincus and Chang, much of Rock's early work consisted of exploring the possibilities of fertilizing eggs in vitro. He also studied and described the entire cycle of human conception and fertilization, from ovulation to embryonic development. Eventually, Rock's work expanded into the treatment of other gynecologic problems, including ectopic pregnancy, cancer of the reproductive organs, pelvic inflammatory disease, endometriosis, and various disorders of menstruation. Despite being a practicing Catholic, Rock was also an ardent supporter of birth control during an era when many states, including Massachusetts, outlawed contraception even for married persons. Rock saw no inconsistencies between his work on infertility and his support for contraception. He believed that the ability to have as many children as one wanted and could reasonably afford—either by seeking treatment for infertility or by limiting the number of births through contraception—was the key to both maternal health and marital happiness. With the exception of the Catholic Church, this opinion was shared by growing numbers of Americans in the postwar era. Although most parents heartily engaged in the baby craze of this period, many also wanted to be able to stop having babies once they had the desired number of children. In 1947, Rock became a founding member of the National Research Council's Committee on Human Reproduction, an endeavor supported by both the National Committee on Maternal Health and Planned Parenthood Federation of America. It was Rock's work on finding substances that could both promote and limit fertility that brought him in touch with the work of Pincus and Chang at the WFEB. Rock demonstrated that the administration of estrogen and progesterone could be used to treat some forms of infertility by creating what he called a rebound reaction, which reset a woman's menstrual cycle so that she would be more likely to conceive once she stopped hormone therapy. The same principle of manipulating the female reproductive cycle could also be applied to preventing pregnancy.[16]

If it were not for the intervention of Margaret Sanger, though, the implications of these findings for contraception may never have been realized. As Pincus recalled, his interest in preventing conception through administration of hormones would have remained at the level of "simple curiosity" had Sanger not persuaded him to find a way to use his findings to fulfill her quest for a reliable, female-controlled form of birth control.[17]

Putting Sanger's idea in motion required funding, and that was in short supply in the early 1950s. Although public opinion was shifting in favor of family planning, research on contraceptives still remained controversial. Searle, like other drug companies at this time, was initially reluctant to invest in this line of research because they feared opposition from religious groups and boycotts of other pharmaceutical products should they market a contraceptive pill. Neither the National Science Foundation nor the National Institutes of Health would fund scientific research on contraception. Although Planned Parenthood was extremely interested in Pincus's work, it did not have sufficient funds to adequately support the foundation's research on contraceptives. Fortunately, Sanger's longtime friend and fellow birth control advocate Katherine Dexter McCormick provided critical funding for research leading to the development of the Pill. McCormick was the widow of Stanley McCormick, one of the heirs to the fortune made by International Harvester founder Cyrus McCormick. Stanley had developed schizophrenia shortly after his marriage to Katherine in 1904. Katherine McCormick first came in contact with the Worcester Foundation because of Pincus's affiliation with the Worcester State Hospital for the Mentally Ill. She helped finance the foundation's research on the use of adrenal steroids to treat schizophrenia. When McCormick learned that the foundation was conducting research on birth control, she reestablished her contact with the organization and gave over a million dollars to fund development and testing of the contraceptive pill. Even then, the first limited studies at Rock's clinic were part of his larger work on infertility. When Searle finally agreed to support this work, the company's initial drug application to the FDA in 1957 for the commercial product Enovid was for the treatment of menstrual disorders, not for contraception. Although Pincus's team managed to do some small human studies using nurse volunteers from Boston hospitals and female psychiatric patients at Worcester State Hospital, in order to conduct a larger study the effectiveness of this drug as a contraceptive, Pincus had to look beyond Massachusetts, where birth control was still illegal.[18]

The ethics of the field trials of oral contraceptives in Puerto Rico and Haiti have been discussed extensively by other historians. These scholars have convincingly demonstrated that concerns about overpopulation among poor people of color were central to the motivations of contraceptive researchers in the 1950s. Both Pincus and Chang, for example, wrote that they became interested in finding new contraceptive methods because of numerous reports of a population explosion in the developing world following the Second World War. Rock, too, argued that the Pill was a natural way to prevent overpopulation because it imitated normal hormonal changes.[19]

The selection of developing regions as laboratories for drug trials also reflected prevailing standards for research involving human subjects. The trials of Nazi physicians following the Second World War had established the Nuremberg Code, stipulating a set of standards regarding ethical treatment of human subjects, but the impact of these new rules on American medical research was uneven. The American Medical Association (AMA) issued a set of research standards that incorporated key principles of the Nuremberg

Code, most notably the need for voluntary, informed consent of research subjects. Yet the AMA standards were vague about what amount of information should be imparted to the research subject and who, if anyone, should oversee human subject research. The AMA standards also said little about the ethics of conducting research on socially disadvantaged individuals in the United States and abroad. The most egregious example of an American research project left untouched by the Nuremberg Code was the Tuskegee study of untreated syphilis in the African American male, which began under the auspices of the American Public Health Service in the 1930s. The study continued until Senate hearings on the treatment of human subjects during the early 1970s brought a halt to this research and other projects that had failed to obtain voluntary informed consent of their subjects.[20]

Yet the field trials of the Pill would not have succeeded without the willing cooperation of female subjects. Healthcare workers in Puerto Rico and Haiti were soon overwhelmed with appeals from women who begged to join the clinical studies. Over eight hundred women enrolled in the field trials in Puerto Rico and Haiti. Although a few women dropped out because of side effects, the majority remained because they desperately wanted a way to prevent unwanted pregnancies. When news about the field trials first appeared in American newspapers and magazines, Pincus received letters from women around the United States eager to volunteer as test subjects for the new contraceptive. The clinical trials convinced the FDA that Enovid was safe, and in May 1960 the agency approved use of the drug for contraceptive purposes in the United States.[21]

Before long, the Pill became the most widely used form of birth control in this country. The rapid adoption of the Pill by American women was fostered by promotional materials distributed to private physicians by pharmaceutical companies. Although direct-to-consumer drug advertising was prohibited, women learned about the Pill via extensive media coverage in popular magazines and newspapers. Planned Parenthood medical director Mary S. Calderone negotiated with drug companies to allow clinics to buy birth control pills at cost and pass the savings along to clinic patients. Within five years of approval, six and a half million married women were taking the Pill. Hundreds of thousands of unmarried women took the pill too, although precisely how many is impossible to determine because they were not included in official reports. Pill use was especially high among young, white, non-Catholic, married, college-educated women: a survey conducted in 1965 indicated 80 percent of women from this category aged twenty to twenty-four had used oral contraceptives.[22]

Sanger's dream of a magic pill that would empower women by granting them full control over their fertility was only partially fulfilled. Although she and McCormick supported research on the Pill because of their interest in women's rights, none of the scientists shared their feminist commitment to reproductive freedom for women. Rock saw the development of reliable contraception as a way to foster marital happiness. He even struggled in vain to convince the Catholic Church that the contraceptive pill was consistent with church doctrine regarding marital relations and fertility control. According to Rock, because the Pill inhibited ovulation, it extended the infertile period that served as the theological basis for the rhythm method approved by the church. The Catholic Church did not agree. In his encyclical *Humanae Vitae* (1968), Pope Paul VI reaffirmed the church's traditional opposition to both abortion and artificial forms of birth control.[23]

Pincus and Chang shared Rock's opinions on family planning as an aid to traditional marriage, not a means of women's liberation. They were also interested in using contraception as a means of alleviating poverty in the United States and the developing world. As Chang wrote years later, finding a scientific solution to world population growth had created great opportunities for experts in reproductive science.[24]

In short, the fathers of the Pill saw unwanted pregnancy as a "disease" that could be cured through advances in scientific research. In the United States, unplanned pregnancies within marriage led to family discord, while "illegitimate" pregnancies outside of wedlock contributed to social problems among the nation's growing numbers of poor people of color. Unchecked population growth in developing countries led to social unrest and political upheaval in these regions. Even Sanger and McCormick shared this disease-based model of contraception. Yet both also believed that by funding scientific research on birth control, they could alleviate the scourge of unwanted pregnancy that limited women's freedoms within and outside of marriage.[25]

Some historians have viewed Sanger's collaboration with the medical professionals as a betrayal of Sanger's earlier commitment to grassroots feminist birth control activism. They have also rightly criticized Sanger for tacitly endorsing the population movement's tendency to focus their efforts on poor people of color in the United States and developing countries.[26] However, Sanger's work also needs to be placed in the larger history of consumer protection in the twentieth century. This consumer movement was led by women who had a major stake in convincing the medical profession and the federal government to protect the public health from dangerous food additives, drugs, and other consumer products. Consumer activism by women's groups played an instrumental role in the passage of the Pure Food and Drug Act in 1906 and the Food, Drug, and Cosmetic Act of 1938. Under the 1938 law, drug manufacturers had to apply to the FDA for approval of new drugs. Further, they had to demonstrate that new drugs were safe for use through extensive pre-market testing.[27]

In an editorial in her *Birth Control Review,* Sanger demonstrated her commitment to protecting women from unscientific and questionable information about contraception. Sanger argued that many women in need of reliable information on birth control were illiterate or poorly educated, and giving these women written information was "like offering a printed bill-of-fare to a starving man." Sanger argued that her approach was more effective because it would allow direct contact between women needing advice and "those competent to teach scientific practical birth control and sex hygiene," that is, "physicians, nurses, and midwives in public and private practice."[28] Nevertheless Sanger's collaboration with physicians reinforced the notion that pregnancy was a disease that needed to be treated with technological solutions developed by medical scientists. This approach to pregnancy prevention, and the racial class biases embedded within it, would shape contraceptive research and development for decades to come.

Prejudice against the Pill

The disease model of contraception was reinforced by the fact that the Pill was available only by prescription. Prior to the Pill's approval by FDA, Congress had passed the Durham-Humphrey Amendment—aka the Prescription Drug Amendment—to the Food, Drug, and Cosmetic Act. Enacted in 1951, this amendment for the first time made a clear distinction between "legend" drugs—that is, those that could only be used under the supervision of a physician—and over-the-counter (OTC) drugs that did not require a prescription. This law made it illegal to give legend drugs to anyone who did not have a valid prescription.[29] In many states, doctors would only prescribe the Pill to married women. Prior to the U.S. Supreme Court decision *Griswold v. Connecticut* (1965), some states considered contraception to be an "offense against Decency, Morality, and Humanity" even within marriage. The *Griswold* decision declared that "Connecticut's birth-control law unconstitutionally intrudes upon the right of marital privacy."[30] The *Griswold* decision said nothing about unmarried individuals, however, and in the wake of this decision some states passed laws explicitly forbidding anyone from providing contraceptives to unmarried persons.[31] In an article for *Esquire* magazine entitled "The Moral Disarmament of Betty Coed" (1962), Gloria Steinem described the various ways in which single women managed to circumvent these restrictions. Some were able to find physicians willing to prescribe the Pill to them, either as a contraceptive or more often for treating menstrual disorders. Others borrowed wedding rings from friends.[32] Yet, these options varied from state to state. In 1967, the Boston vice squad arrested contraceptive salesman Bill Baird for "crimes against chastity" after he gave a can of spermicidal foam to an unmarried teenaged girl following a lecture at Boston University.[33]

Medical literature on the Pill and advertising to physicians reinforced the notion that this drug was meant to enhance marital relations, not sexually liberate unmarried women. Although some psychiatrists worried that eliminating the fear of pregnancy would cause men to be dominated by sexually aggressive women, most agreed that freedom from unwanted births would draw couples closer together and prevent the family discord and economic distress that often accompanied excessive childbearing.[34]

Soon after the release of the Pill, reports began appearing in the popular media about the possible side effects of the drug. Most articles focused on minor side effects, such as headache, nausea, bloating, and weight gain. However, some also reported on the rare cases of women who had suffered blood clots and other serious side complications while taking oral contraceptives.[35] These reports appeared shortly after horrifying news about birth defects caused by thalidomide, a sedative administered to pregnant women to reduce morning sickness. The drug had not received approval in the United States due to the strict regulations imposed by the Food, Drug, and Cosmetic Act of 1938. The FDA's refusal to approve thalidomide in the United States both enhanced the image of the agency and led to calls for even tighter regulations for the approval of new drugs. In 1962, Congress passed the Kefauver-Harris amendments to the 1938 Food, Drug, and Cosmetic Act. These amendments required that manufacturers prove that a new drug was both safe and effective in treating the condition for which it was administered. Pharmaceutical companies also had to include both the risks and benefits of drugs in all advertising to physicians, and they still could not directly advertise their products to consumers.[36]

Although the Pill was approved for use prior to the 1962 amendments, in response to reports of serious side effects among some users, the FDA issued a statement pronouncing the Pill was safe only for short-term use (two to four years) in women under the age of thirty-five. The FDA also requested that Searle send a letter to physicians warning them that blood clotting was a possible side effect of pill use.[37]

Federal law did not require that this information be provided directly to women through a patient package insert, but these dangers were widely reported in the popular press. Although Planned Parenthood and other family planning organizations tried to stem the growing tide of negative publicity regarding the Pill, polls conducted in the mid to late 1960s indicated that negative reports had significantly affected women's attitudes toward use of the Pill. A Gallup poll conducted in 1966 indicated that 43 percent of women considered the Pill was safe, 26 percent said it was not, and 31 percent had no opinion. Three years later, only 22 percent considered the Pill to be safe, 46 percent thought it unsafe, and 32 percent were unsure.[38]

Some commentators stated this backlash against the Pill was excessive. In an article for the popular women's magazine *McCall's,* entitled "Why Birth Control Fails" (1969), Lawrence Lader criticized the "prejudice against the Pill" among highly educated women: only 11 percent reported they used this method of contraception. Lader claimed these women not only were misinformed, but "frighteningly irresponsible about birth control and are ignorant enough to use methods like rhythm and withdrawal, which hardly deserve to be ranked as contraception."[39] Psychiatrists conducted studies of the alleged side effects reported by women who took oral contraceptives, hoping to discern whether these symptoms were physiological or psychological in origin. In most cases, they argued that most minor side effects were caused by guilt about using birth control and ambivalence about trying to prevent a pregnancy.[40]

Consumers were not the only ones who had concerns about the Pill's limitations: physicians tended to view white, middle-class women as the only ones who were capable of being reliable users of this product. Some argued that even well-educated women could be sabotaged by unconscious wishes and desires. In an article in *Ladies' Home Journal* published in 1965, Barbara Seaman explored the psychological issues that lay behind many failed attempts to prevent pregnancy. Although some doctors gave examples of men who subconsciously thwarted efforts at family planning because they wanted to prove their masculinity or get back at their wives, Seaman observed that "more often, the accident-prone partner in the unplanned pregnancy is the woman." One psychoanalyst argued that a woman who had a "competitive or belittling mother" might find it difficult to defer her first pregnancy. Such a woman could not "feel her mother's equal in femininity until she had a baby too." Other "deeply emotional" causes of unplanned pregnancies included premenopausal panic, marital infidelity, impeding divorce, and other marital stresses. All of these could lead to an "emotional desire for pregnancy that is neither conscious nor rationally sound."[41]

In the case of less-educated women, especially poor women of color, physicians believed intrauterine devices were more suitable for contraception than the Pill because this technology did not rely on the sustained motivation of the user. This philosophy also reflected the economic realities of poor women's lives. Before the creation of Medicaid, the considerable cost of contraceptive pills put them beyond the reach of low-income women who lacked health insurance. The advantage of an IUD was that it involved only the cost of the device and of the doctor's visit for insertion, rather than the ongoing expense of monthly packages of contraceptive pills. During the mid-1960s, access to contraception became a key component of the anti-poverty programs instituted during the administration of President Lyndon Johnson. In addition to Medicaid, Johnson's War on Poverty included the creation of federally funded family planning clinics for low-income women. Some civil rights activists supported these efforts, viewing access to family planning services as a key component of poor women's right to healthcare. African American women in particular argued that they deserved the same access to reliable birth control as white women. However, more radical groups, such as the Nation of Islam, claimed that federal family planning programs were part of a genocidal, white plot against people of color. Even supporters of birth control observed that women of color were more likely to be involuntarily sterilized as part of attempts to control U.S. population growth.[42] Thus, the potentially liberating powers of the Pill were confined to a narrow segment of American women, and even they were becoming increasingly disenchanted with this birth control method.

The Double Life of Estrogen

In order to deal with the failed promises of the Pill, scientists searched for new methods that would compensate for user error and also reduce the cost of contraception to the individual user. During the late 1950s and 1960s, Chang continued to perform studies of chemical compounds that affected fertilization following coitus and artificial insemination. Chang not only found that certain estrogens and progesterones prevented fertilization by reducing sperm capacitation, he also showed that administration of these compounds accelerated the transport of eggs through the reproductive tracts of rats and rabbits, making it less likely that these eggs would be fertilized and implanted in the uterus. Progesterone worked better if administered before ovulation, while estrogen worked better if administered after ovulation.[43] Chang believed that his discoveries had major implications for the "so-called population explosion" and suggested that effective "'morning-after pills,' 'week later pills,' 'second-thought pills,' 'abortion pills' or 'night before pills'" would be developed in the near future. Such breakthroughs, he said, "would be a boon for couples who wanted 100 percent effectiveness in preventing pregnancy." These "after-the-fact" forms of contraception would also be helpful for developing countries, "where contraceptive use was less than perfect, for even a small reduction in the birth rate could alleviate the problems of overpopulation."[44]

Pincus and Chang soon began a small-scale clinical investigation on women at several Boston area hospitals to test the impact of the new technique in humans. Both scientists believed that postcoital contraception offered certain advantages over the ordinary birth control pill regimen. In addition to offering a back-up when a woman failed to start a twenty-pill cycle on time, they argued, the new pill was also less expensive than other birth control pills. The new pill also addressed emerging debates about the safety of hormonal contraception. According to Chang, "it is always better to reach a specific target than the whole system." Since the hormonal impact of a morning-after pill was transitory, he argued, it was possibly safer than conventional oral contraceptives.[45] Pincus and Chang's work on the postcoital pill caused a major split with Rock, who believed that the new pill was virtually an abortifacient and therefore inconsistent with Catholic doctrine.[46]

The WFEB did not pursue work on the morning-after pill for long. Pincus died in 1967. Chang returned his attention to perfecting methods of in vitro fertilization.[47] It was left to other researchers to expand upon their work. The first to follow up on Chang's findings in the United States were John McLean Morris and Gertrude van Wagenen in the Department of Obstetrics and Gynecology at the Yale University School of Medicine. Morris observed, "Recent publicity concerning thalidomide has focused attention on the role of drugs taken during pregnancy." Morris soon began work on exploring other teratogens (substances that caused fetal defects). He was particular interested in exploring the causes of intersex conditions. He found that some babies with female chromosomes would acquire male characteristics if exposed to high doses of certain hormones while in utero.[48]

Like other medical researchers who entered the field of contraceptive innovation at this time, Morris believed that the "most important problem before the medical profession today is the problem of population control."[49] Building on the work of Pincus and Chang, Morris and van Wagenen performed the first tests of postcoital contraception in primates, using van Wagenen's macaque monkey colony as subjects. [50] They noted that any substance used for this purpose had to be nontoxic, 100 percent effective, and harmless to a fetus should the subject turn out to be pregnant when given the drug. The first compound they used was ORF-3858, a carbolic acid derivative developed by Ortho Pharmaceuticals in New Jersey. Because this drug did not yet have FDA approval, Morris and van Wagenen had to find a commercially available drug before they could extend their tests to humans. Because estrogen had shown the most promise in other animal studies, they looked for a suitable drug product manufactured and sold in the United States for their experiments.[51]

By the mid-1960s, there were a variety of estrogen products from which to choose. In addition to contraceptive pills, pharmaceutical companies had developed estrogen compounds to treat a number of gynecological disorders and complications of pregnancy. These included Ethinyl, a hormone replacement product manufactured by Shering; the pregnancy test Gestest, produced by Squibb; and the non-steroidal, synthetic estrogen diethylstilbestrol (DES), created by Eli Lilly. Although Morris and van Wagenen acknowledged any estrogen substance in sufficient doses could be effective as a postcoital contraceptive, they eventually chose to use DES because it was more potent than any other estrogen compound. Therefore, it could be administered in smaller doses and minimize side effects such as nausea and vomiting that often accompanied oral ingestion of high doses of estrogen. DES was also cheaper to produce in large quantities because it could be easily manufactured from coal tar. Because the other scientists who discovered DES were financed by the British Medical Research Council, they were not permitted to patent the compound. The low cost of production, therefore, made DES attractive to many pharmaceutical companies in both Britain and the United States.[52]

DES was one of the first drugs approved under the new, more rigorous standards imposed by the U.S. Food, Drug, and Cosmetic Act of 1938. In May 1941, a consortium of twelve pharmaceutical firms submitted a new drug application (NDA) to the FDA for approval of DES. The manufacturers did not have to demonstrate that DES was effective: that requirement only came with Kefauver-Harris amendments to the law in 1962. Although a significant number of users experienced nausea and vomiting while taking DES, the FDA found that these side effects were not serious enough to decline the NDA. In September 1941 the FDA approved sale of DES in the United States for treatment of gonorrheal vaginitis, menopausal symptoms, and suppression of lactation. In 1947, several drug companies applied for a supplemental drug application after tests showed the drug might be effective in treating high-risk pregnancies. The FDA approved the supplemental drug application and in 1952 declared that because DES had been proven to be safe, drug manufacturers no longer needed to get FDA approval to market the drug for other purposes.[53]

Although FDA was in charge of approving new drugs, it could not oversee the prescribing habits of physicians. Hence, it was not uncommon for physicians to use prescription drugs off-label for conditions other than those for which they had originally received FDA approval. The general science journal *Science News* announced in 1967 that DES and other estrogens could have a "double-life" as both treatments for reproductive disorders and as morning-after pills. Although FDA prohibited drug companies from advertising or recommending that estrogens be used postcoitally, private physicians could prescribe them as they saw fit, since FDA regulated the drug industry, not the practice of medicine.[54] The way was cleared for researchers to explore further uses of DES in humans. All that was needed was a group of human volunteers on which to test the effectiveness of the drug as a morning-after pill.

Chapter 2

Courageous Volunteers

In 1966, John McLean Morris and Gertrude van Wagenen reported the results of their first human tests of postcoital contraception at the Annual Meeting of the American Gynecological Society. Morris and Van Wagenen noted that despite the success of their studies in the macaque monkey, they were initially anxious about extending their research to human beings because the risk of side effects in humans was unknown. Their first human subjects were rape victims treated at Yale–New Haven Hospital. Morris and van Wagenen acknowledged that the incidence of pregnancy following rape was uncertain. They found that none of their small sample of patients became pregnant. Side effects were rare and, when they occurred, consisted chiefly of nausea and breast tenderness that ceased after medication was stopped. The researchers then solicited a small number of what they called "courageous volunteers," consisting of married female graduate students and faculty wives at Yale University who agreed to serve as additional test subjects for the drug. These preliminary trials also resulted in no pregnancies, but given the small number of subjects, they concluded, "these results should be viewed with caution."[1]

In his discussion of Morris and van Wagenen's presentation, Somer Sturgis, professor of gynecology at Harvard Medical School, suggested that Morris and van Wagenen's work "may be the most important advance in antifertility research in the human being since the pathfinding work of Rock and Pincus more than a decade ago." Indeed, Sturgis found it even more significant since the problem of overpopulation in economically deprived regions could not be solved by the standard birth control regimen of daily pills for twenty-four days of the menstrual cycle. "Yet the coital act itself can be universally accepted as a signal to take medication to prevent conception by the most primitive of peoples," Sturgis argued.[2] Thus, controlling world population growth should be the ultimate goal of Morris and van Wagenen's studies.

Charles E. McLennan of the Department of Obstetrics and Gynecology at Stanford University Medical School expressed his hope that the research team would soon be able to locate even more "courageous volunteers, seduced or otherwise, to give him the real answers on mode of action, dosage, and timing." Indeed, said McLennan, "the supply of experimental subjects might become relatively enormous if campus vending machines could dispense little 'six-packs' of stilbestrol tablets, each packet promising a refund if the user would simply report results promptly to a central registry in New Haven." However, McLennan noted, "no doubt the FDA would veto such a straightforward approach to science."[3]

These statements reflect the race and class biases that shaped contraceptive research and development in the United States. Advances in birth control technology were viewed as a way to "cure" the "disease" of unwanted pregnancy among poor people of color both domestically and in the developing world. McLennan's flip comments about campus vending machines reveal the era's discomfort with the changing sexual practices of the nation's college students, especially those of young women. In both cases, postcoital contraception was touted as a panacea for the consequences of uncontrolled female sexuality. Although no one took McLennan's remarks literally, it was "courageous volunteers" like those at Yale who served as subjects for these further studies of the morning-after pill.

Birth Control Is Booming in the Elm City

Yale–New Haven Hospital was at the center of birth control politics in both the state of Connecticut and the nation as a whole. Dr. C. Lee Buxton, chair of Yale Medical School's Department of Obstetrics and Gynecology, and Planned Parenthood League of Connecticut executive director Estelle Griswold of the city's Planned Parenthood chapter were the lead plaintiffs in the landmark *Griswold v. Connecticut* U.S. Supreme Court decision. In 1958, Buxton and three of his patients filed a lawsuit claiming that the state's laws prohibiting the sale, distribution, and use of contraceptive drugs and devices were unconstitutional. The suit reached the U.S. Supreme Court in June of 1961, but the Court dismissed the case since no state laws had been violated. Yet, the Court opinion that accompanied the decision also declared Connecticut laws were "dead words and harmless, empty shadows." On November 1 of that year, the Planned Parenthood League of Connecticut (PPLC), led by

Estelle Griswold, decided to test the validity of the court's opinion and opened a birth control clinic in New Haven. Nine days later Buxton and Griswold were arrested for violating state laws outlawing contraception. The defendants appealed their case all the way to the U.S. Supreme Court, culminating in the court's decision in *Griswold v. Connecticut* (1965), declaring that Connecticut's birth-control law unconstitutionally intruded upon the right of marital privacy.[4]

Immediately following the *Griswold* decision, the Connecticut Birth Control League opened the New Haven Planned Parenthood clinic. Initially, league officials reported an uphill battle in gaining acceptance for their work due to a lingering moral stigma against family planning. By 1967, the situation had changed dramatically: the *Yale Daily News* proclaimed that "birth control is booming in the Elm City." In the words of one PPLC volunteer, "everyone is getting on the bandwagon," including female graduate students at Yale University, which at that time still did not admit women to the undergraduate college. According to the league's executive director, Donald Tall, Yale women used the clinic because it was close to campus and because the Yale University Health Service did not provide birth control nor did it have a gynecologist on staff. Instead the Yale University Health Service referred female students to Planned Parenthood or private doctors. The *Yale Daily News* reported that the Planned Parenthood clinic would serve any woman over the age of twenty-one (the age of majority at that time), even if she was not married. Although Connecticut did not mandate parental consent for unmarried minors to receive birth control, leaving this up to the discretion of the provider or clinic, Planned Parenthood required single minors have the written consent of a parent in order to receive services.[5] The same was true of unmarried minors who sought services at Yale–New Haven Hospital.[6]

The life-altering consequences of these restrictions on the care of minors would spur further use of the morning-after pill at Yale–New Haven Hospital. Morris's work was part of a larger initiative by the obstetrics and gynecology program to address the city's growing problem of unwed teenage motherhood. The problem of teenage pregnancy was not unique to New Haven. Despite the declining age of marriage following the Second World War, the rate of births to unmarried adolescent girls in the United States tripled between 1940 and 1957. Views about how to address this problem were strongly shaped by racial biases. During the 1950s and early 1960s, physicians tended to believe unwed pregnancy among black teenagers was due to the allegedly greater tolerance of illegitimacy among African Americans. White girls who became pregnant out of wedlock, in contrast, were depicted as neurotic or maladjusted, particularly if they insisted on keeping their babies without marrying the father. Medical experts claimed that the "cure" for a white unwed mother's psychological problems was to convince her to either legitimize her pregnancy by marrying the child's father or give up the baby for adoption and prepare for a "normal" path to marriage and motherhood.[7]

By the mid-1960s, some experts suggested that helping girls of color to complete their educations would help alleviate the social and economic consequences of teenage pregnancy in these groups. In 1963, the U.S. Children's Bureau began funding the Webster School Project for pregnant school-aged girls in the District of Columbia. The first full-time public school of pregnant adolescents in the United States, the Webster School combined education, healthcare, and counseling for personal problems. Researchers associated with the Webster School showed that their approach significantly improved the educational attainment and career opportunities for girls who attended the school. Other cities created similar programs: by the mid-1960s there were nearly forty projects serving eight thousand pregnant teenagers around the country.[8]

In 1965, the Obstetrics and Gynecology Department at Yale–New Haven Hospital created the Young Mothers program, which was modeled after the Webster School project. Like other programs, the one at Yale–New Haven hoped to disrupt the cycle of poverty that contributed to the population crisis and the growth of a permanent nonwhite underclass. The Yale researchers noted with pride their ability to help their clients become "productive human beings" rather than reproductive ones. Although the staff of the Young Mothers program focused on African American girls, they also argued that unwed teenage pregnancy was a problem among white teenagers as well. They observed that white girls were more likely to be delivered by private physicians or in homes for unwed mothers. They also speculated that white girls had greater access to physicians willing to prescribe oral contraceptives to unmarried minors even without parental consent. Therefore, a key component of the Young Mothers program was to provide postpartum contraception to their young patients, but only if their parents gave consent to do so.[9]

These physicians were motivated not only by the problem of "recidivism"—that is, repeat pregnancies among teenaged mothers they attended—but also by a marked increase in the number of young women who came to the hospital in septic shock from illegal abortions. Like most states at this time, Connecticut had very strict abortion laws. Yale–New Haven provided abortions only after a hospital committee determined that pregnancy posed a risk to a woman's life or her mental or physical health. White, middle-class girls were more likely to have the financial resources to travel to states with less restrictive abortion laws and thus had better access to safe abortions. Low-income women were less fortunate and frequently wound up suffering serious complications or dying of blood loss or infection following unsafe abortion procedures.[10]

Physicians at Yale–New Haven also began to recognize that incest and rape were contributing factors in the cycle of unwed pregnancy in disadvantaged social groups.[11] Prior to the mid-1960s, physicians tended to ignore the problem of sexual abuse of children and adolescents. Pediatricians who treated sexually transmitted diseases in their young patients insisted that these infections were acquired from innocent sources such as toilet seats that had been contaminated with infectious material. Physicians were especially likely to use these modes of transmission to explain cases in which the family was white, well-to-do, and socially prominent. Even when the family was from a lower socioeconomic group, child and adolescent cases of venereal disease were usually attributed to the alleged filth and squalor of most lower-class homes, rather than to sexual abuse by family members. Pediatricians and gynecologists seldom learned how to perform pelvic exams on girls and young women: in fact, the practice was actively discouraged by most pediatric and gynecological textbooks. Physicians were therefore ill-equipped to recognize the signs of sexual abuse in girls and young women.[12]

The criminal justice system was even less helpful to women and girls who were victims of sexual assault. During the first half of the twentieth century, legal discussions of rape tended to focus on the psychopathology of the perpetrator rather than the mental health needs of the victim. Mental health professionals argued that rapists suffered from a character disorder and argued that these individuals needed medical treatment not punishment. At the same time, psychologists and sexologists argued that female sexual pleasure was both normal and desirable. This had the unintended conse-quence of reframing rape as a crime in which women played a role in their own victimization by tempting men who were unable to control their sexual impulses. In other words, many believed that women who were raped had provoked their attacker by behaving in a sexual provocative manner. Rape laws allowed the victim's prior sexual history to be admitted as evidence during criminal proceedings, effectively putting women on trial along with their abusers.[13]

During the mid-1960s, rape victims and their supporters began to chal-lenge these views. In 1965, a woman who had been raped in the District of Columbia complained bitterly to the local and national press about the inhumane treatment she received from law enforcement and emergency medical personnel. The victim reported that police treated her more like a "cold statistic than a human being," holding her for three hours of questioning before taking her to the hospital. She then waited nearly two hours in the emergency room before being examined by a physician, who did not offer her any methods to prevent pregnancy. Eventually, the fed-up patient went to a private physician who treated her more than seven hours after the initial assault. This scandal prompted the District's public health department to improve treatment for sexually assaulted females. They were especially intent on helping children and adolescents from lower socioeconomic levels who did not have access to a family physician.[14] Still, in many states, unmarried patients under age twenty-one had to receive permission from a parent or guardian before they could receive contraceptive pills or devices.[15]

One way around laws regulating minors' access to birth control was to use a provision in the law that allowed for treatment of minors without parental consent when a case was considered an emergency. Morris believed sexual assault cases fit these criteria and underscored the significance of the morning-after pill for the young rape victims he saw at Yale–New Haven Hospital: "It means that the girl who has been raped and has a good chance of becoming pregnant doesn't have to worry," he said, because she will "know that there is available retroactive contraception."[16]

Other urban hospitals soon adopted this back-up method of birth control for the treatment of rape victims. In 1967, a group of physicians in the Obstetrics and Gynecology Department at Pennsylvania General Hospital began a study of the effectiveness of postcoital contraceptive therapy in preventing pregnancy in sexually assaulted girls and women. One of the principal investigators in the study was Dr. Celso-Ramon Garcia, chief of obstetrics and gynecology at the University of Pennsylvania, who had collaborated with Pincus and Rock on the field trials for the first contraceptive pill. Garcia and his colleagues shared many of the era's preconceptions about rape victims, arguing that even the child victim could be a willing participant in the sexual act. Although they recognized the psychological and social consequences of rape, these researchers were mainly interested in preventing the most serious side effect of sexual assault—unwanted pregnancy. Nevertheless, these researchers did recognize the importance of informed consent and warned their subjects in writing that postcoital use of DES to prevent pregnancy was experimental and could have unknown side effects.[17] Meanwhile, the team at

Yale–New Haven began to address the needs of a new population in need of after-the-fact contraception: female undergraduates at Yale.

Sex and the Yale Student

Like other elite male colleges during the late 1960s, Yale decided to admit women to the undergraduate college in the fall of 1969. In the buildup to coeducation, the University Health Service (UHS) recognized it had to provide reproductive healthcare to female students and hired assistant professor of obstetrics and gynecology Phillip Sarrel to serve as staff gynecologist. They also hired Sarrel's wife, Lorna, a social worker, to help him develop a sex counseling service for both female and male students within the Mental Health Division of the UHS.[18]

The Sarrels began working with college students in western Massachusetts in 1967, offering informal sex education classes at Mount Holyoke, Smith, Amherst, and the University of Massachusetts. At this time, the Commonwealth of Massachusetts still considered it a "crime against chastity" to give birth control to unmarried individuals. During the two years they worked the Five College region, the Sarrels were part of a network of sympathetic healthcare professionals, faculty, and clergy who helped young women circumvent the Commonwealth's restrictive contraception and abortion laws. They therefore were a natural choice for the new gynecological and sex counseling service at Yale.[19]

The day before fall classes started, the Sarrels gave an overview of the new service to a gathering of female students. The *Yale Daily News* reported that the purpose of the service was "not to moralize" and that the staff considered the question "are you married" to be irrelevant. At the same time, the paper warned that the service would not function simply as dispensary for birth control pills. Instead, students would "discuss their sexual needs with the Sarrels and various methods of solving their problems." The Sarrels hoped not only to provide birth control but "to help students face the tremendous sexual pressures of the college environment." They were especially concerned that many young women were "getting involved in relationships they don't really want, and are not really ready for, but are getting involved in because of social pressures here."[20]

Within six months, the *Yale Daily News* reported that the service was so popular that there was a two-month wait for appointments, although women who needed urgent care were seen immediately. In emergency cases involving unprotected intercourse, Dr. Sarrel prescribed a morning-after pill. In non-urgent cases, he recommended a trip to the local drugstore, adding that many students were not aware that reliable methods of birth control were available over the counter. He concluded that there was a much lower pregnancy rate than he originally predicted when Yale went coed, a fact he attributed to "the responsible sexual behavior of Yale students."[21]

This conscientiousness owed much to the organizational efforts of students. Interest in advice on sexual matters was so great that the Sarrels enlisted the help of student leaders on campus to help coordinate a noncredit Topics in Human Sexuality course, modeled after ones that the Sarrels had conducted at Smith College and Brown University. The course consisted of lectures by Dr. Sarrel and Amherst College psychology professor Haskell Coplin, followed by discussion groups led by undergraduate students. First offered in spring 1970, the Yale course attracted over one thousand students, which made it the largest course in Yale history and the largest sex education course on the East Coast at that time. The *Yale Daily News* reported that most of the students in the course were undergraduates, and 20 percent of the students in the course were women, even though only 12 percent of the Yale student body was female.[22]

One of the texts selected by the student coordinating committee to use in the human sexuality course was the *Birth Control Handbook,* developed by students at McGill University in Montreal in 1968 and financed by student councils at ten Canadian universities, Princeton University, and the University of Maine. The McGill handbook criticized the American-led population movement, especially the organization Zero Population Growth (ZPG), which they called a right-wing, eugenicist organization that used birth control as a "genocidal weapon" against the non-white peoples of the world.[23] The Yale student committee in charge of coordinating the human sexuality course inserted a disclaimer in the copies of the McGill handbook used in the human sexuality course, disavowing the handbooks contention "that capitalist countries are using birth control as a form of genocide to oppress the underdeveloped nations."[24]

Yale students soon developed their own self-help guide, entitled *Sex and the Yale Student* (1970), which they touted as a "*Yale* pamphlet, by and for Yale students, and centered on our concerns and our questions about human sexuality." The student editors hoped that they would reach all Yale students, not just those who attended the human sexuality course. The guide explained that, unlike most universities, Yale had a health service that would provide birth control to students. The policy of the gynecological service was to "individualize each case" so that "each student understands the limitations of all methods of birth control and that the student is aware of any problems that might develop." The pamphlet gave detailed information about recent reports on rare major complications, such as blood clots and strokes. The book also had a section on the morning-after pill, offering encouraging news: "If something goes wrong with your contraceptive program (assuming you have some contraceptive program!)—perhaps you forgot to take your pill or maybe your condom burst or came off . . . or if you have had unprotected intercourse, there is something you can do to avoid a possible pregnancy!" The guide stated that the health service set aside special appointment times so that that students requesting post-intercourse contraception could be seen at those times. The book noted side effects—nausea and vomiting—but said "most people feel that this is a small price to pay for the reduction of anxiety or the prevention of pregnancy." Yet it also warned, "because of the high estrogen content, the morning after pill should be used *only* as a back-up method and not as a method of contraception."[25]

Yale was one of the few institutions of higher education to offer birth control in the student health service at this time. A survey conducted by the American College Health Association in 1970 indicated that only 118 institutions offered contraceptive services. This represented a fraction of the over 2,500 colleges and universities in the United States at that time. Although the reasons for these statistics were not stated, it is possible that fear of prosecution played a role in the dearth of birth control services offered at college and university health centers.[26] A more powerful disincentive, of course, was concern about the impact that offering contraceptive services would have on state funding and alumni donations. As one recent graduate of Mills College in California sardonically told *Glamour* magazine in 1970, "If Mills came out strong for birth control, some little old lady in Menlo Park might decide this is just a bit much from her old alma mater and withhold her yearly check."[27]

Sarrel also blamed the lack of campus birth control services on physicians' tendency to think of contraception for teenagers and young adults as mainly a problem among the poor. He reported that his interviews with students indicated that "college students are not promiscuous, but that they are often ignorant and unrealistic about their behavior. Frequently girls refuse to face the fact that they are not 'immune' to pregnancy." He argued that on-campus access to contraception could prevent major disasters, such as a girl who may become pregnant from her first sexual exposure. He also stated that campus health services should provide psychological support as well as contraception, especially in cases of sexual assault or other incidences of unprotected intercourse. Dr. Sarrel urged his colleagues at other institutions not to "hide behind the law. . . . If it is good medical practice to prevent a girl from becoming pregnant . . . then the law should be circumvented so that the girl does not go to a criminal abortionist."[28]

The Morning-After Pill Gets Around

Students on other campuses followed Yale's example by creating their own self-help guides. The Boston University Student Congress published a pamphlet on birth control, abortion, and venereal disease as an "act of civil disobedience" against the Boston police. These students, most of whom were women, worked closely with feminist organizations in Boston and Cambridge and held public demonstrations demanding reproductive rights for women.[29] At nearby Radcliffe College, the private women's college affiliated with Harvard University, students complained that when they went to the college health service for contraceptive advice, doctors made them feel guilty or abnormal.[30] To meet the need for accurate knowledge, Radcliffe students put together their own guide to birth control providers in the Boston area.[31] During the late 1960s and early 1970s, dozens of other self-help publications appeared on campuses and college towns throughout the country.[32]

Male students played an important role in this contraceptive self-help movement. James Trussell, an undergraduate at all-male Davidson College in Charlotte, North Carolina, began offering lectures on birth control to his classmates during the late 1960s. Trussell first became interested in population issues as a high school student in Columbus, Georgia. "I saw some of my classmates drop out because of it, and I began to think of how stupid and sad it was that high school students don't know about birth control," he told a reporter from the University of North Carolina student newspaper, the *Daily Tar Heel*. Trussell was soon asked to expand his lectures to include women students at nearby Queens College, under a program called Free University, sponsored by student groups at both Davidson and Queens. Trussell recalled, "There were quite a few girls in my course, some out of curiosity, I think. I suppose some of them were embarrassed at times, but no one was pushed to say anything. There was no forcing."[33] In the summer of 1970, Trussell received a grant from the Institute for the Study of Health and Society, developed by Students of the American Medical Association to give future medical professionals experience working among non-elite populations and in remote rural areas. In the introduction to *The Loving Book,* an advice manual resulting from Trussell's work with the institute, Trussell and co-author Steve Chandler wrote, "We are both college students who have seen the very real need for this type of information in our own schools and communities. It is hoped that those who read this manual will gain a greater insight into their own sexuality."[34]

In addition to offering basic information about contraception and sexuality, these self-help publications raised awareness of the morning-after pill among college and university students. The Boston-area organization Female Liberation published a notice assuring women that "there really is such a thing as a 'morning-after pill,' the only problem is most women don't know about it."[35] These guides were careful to mention that this method was a last resort, not a replacement for more conventional birth control methods. The Boston University handbook warned, "There is not yet enough data to prove its effectiveness and it is not yet on the open market."[36] The University of Washington guide, *How to Have Intercourse without Getting Screwed,* warned of unpleasant side effects such as nausea, vomiting, and breast tenderness. The guide added that the morning-after pill contained extremely high doses of estrogen, "equivalent to taking the pill for forty-one years. Those risks, such as clotting, associated with birth-control pills are present with morning-after pills." Because the physical effects of repeated treatments were unknown, many health facilities were reluctant to give the treatment more than once to the same woman. Therefore, the guide recommended using the morning-after pill only in cases of "extreme emergencies."[37] A handbook for students at SUNY Buffalo listed the morning-after pill under the category "not recommended treatments," arguing that "this treatment is in no way a substitute for conscientious birth control."[38]

Students who could not find birth control on campus sought out such services from sympathetic health professionals in the community. At the University of North Carolina, Chapel Hill, students consulted Dr. Takey Crist, a gynecologist at North Carolina Memorial Hospital and a member of the faculty in the UNC School of Medicine Department of Obstetrics and Gynecology. In 1969, Crist and his colleagues in the medical school conducted a survey of the contraceptive practices of six hundred women at UNC. Crist reported that "while the modern coed may now feel more free to indulge in sexual relations, her ignorance of contraception is appalling" because contraceptives and related sexual information were not available on most college campuses.[39] In order to meet the demand for information at UNC, Crist and undergraduate Lana Starnes started a sex information column in the *Daily Tar Heel,* where they answered questions regarding sex and contraception, as well as more routine hygiene questions such as whether an unmarried girl should use tampons or sanitary napkins. Crist also collaborated with medical students from the University of Chicago, the University of California at Irvine, and the University of South Dakota to produce the advice manual *Elephants and Butterflies . . . and Contraceptives* (1970). The booklet was published and distributed by the

University of North Carolina student Environmental Concerns Committee (ECOS), and "dedicated to the prevention of the tragedy of unwanted pregnancies and venereal disease." The booklet described "morning-after" treatments containing synthetic or natural estrogens that were effective in preventing unwanted pregnancy in cases where the condom tore or when a couple had unprotected intercourse. "If you find yourself in such a predicament," the booklet advised, "you should not panic and, *above all,* you should not douche," but contact the Health Education Clinic or the ob-gyn department at the medical school's Memorial Hospital to request post-intercourse treatment. The booklet noted that "post-intercourse methods should be considered a 'last resort,' to be used after other methods have failed. They are *not* intended as a substitute for regular, conscientious use of the more familiar methods described in previous pages of this booklet."[40] Crist called on other campuses to sponsor similar initiatives to help students prevent unwanted pregnancy, arguing, "It is not our job to establish what is good or bad, but what is necessary."[41]

Elsewhere, students found that local Planned Parenthood affiliates were the best way to gain access to reliable birth control. *Time* magazine reported in 1969 that at Stanford, many of the university's female students were seeking contraceptive help at the nearby Palo Alto Planned Parenthood center.[42] At the University of California at Berkeley, students created a "free-sex movement" alongside Berkeley's infamous Free Speech Movement by distributing birth control literature on the University's Sproul Plaza.[43] Students learned about the morning-after pill from local newspapers. In a 1969 article entitled "A Morning-After Pill for Absent-Minded Lovers," the *San Francisco Chronicle* reported on the perfect solution for the young woman "who has forgotten to take the pill but both she and her boyfriend are feeling especially amorous."[44] University of California students could not find this contraceptive at the University Health Services (UHS). Although UHS director Dr. Henry Bruyn was willing to make birth control information available to students, he did not think that it was the responsibility of the health service to prescribe or distribute contraceptive pills or devices.[45] Consequently, the Planned Parenthood of Alameda County in nearby Oakland, California, found that 60 percent of its caseload consisted of Berkeley students.[46]

In response to student interest in birth control at Berkeley and elsewhere, Planned Parenthood–World Population (PP-WP) initiated the Program of Student Community Action in 1969 and appointed twenty-five-year-old Dan Pellegrom to direct the program. Pellegrom was a recent graduate of the divinity school at Columbia University, where he had served as student government president during the infamous student strike of 1968. Officials at Planned

Parenthood were heartened by the enthusiasm of college students and tried to cultivate a relationship that would encourage a free exchange of ideas and respond to student initiatives rather than dictating them.[47]

Like other initiatives sponsored by Planned Parenthood at this time, the Program of Student Community Action received criticism from a few African American leaders who believed the organization was engaging in "genocide" by targeting poor women of color.[48] In the fall of 1969, Louis Lomax, a black studies professor at Hofstra, alleged that two nineteen-year-old black students had been put in a clinical trial of low-estrogen birth control pills and that black students had complained to Lomax about Planned Parenthood's supposedly aggressive recruitment program on campus. In response, PP-WP affiliates director Naomi Gray, an African American and an emerging leader in the fight for reproductive rights for women of color, agreed to meet with Lomax and other black faculty to discuss the problem.[49]

The results of this meeting are unknown, as is the point of view of the black women at Hofstra. Elsewhere, though, many black female students were at least as adamant as their white counterparts in seeking access to birth control. One study of four thousand college women, white and black, attending institutions in the southeastern United States stated that almost all respondents expected their health services to dispense contraceptives.[50] Planned Parenthood leaders recognized that enlisting the support of black students was essential in establishing the legitimacy of birth control among the African American community, both on and off campus. Douglas Stewart, director of Planned Parenthood's Office of Community Relations and an African American, said that birth control programs might be more successful if Planned Parenthood did a better job of recruiting blacks to serve in the organization. Stewart argued that having a larger black presence in the organization on both the local and national level would go a long way toward counteracting charges of genocide that left many women "caught between pressures from militant groups and their own wishes for fewer children."[51] To achieve this goal, the college program actively encouraged African American students' involvement. One of the earliest college chapters was at Hampton Institute, a historically black college in Virginia.

White students also challenged the racist assumptions of the more extreme population control advocates. James Trussell, for example, said his experience working with impoverished blacks in the Muscogee County, Georgia, Health Department family planning clinics led him to conclude that when all birth control facilities were aimed at poor people of color, it was not difficult to understand why some of them thought contraceptive services were "an attempt at genocide." Trussell argued that the so-called population crisis was mainly a product of the Baby Boom among the college-educated, white middle class. Therefore, family planning providers had to reach this audience as well and convince them that having three or more children was contributing to the population problem in the United States.[52]

At the same time, Planned Parenthood officials showed some qualms with what they considered to be the more politically extreme student organizations, particularly those representing radical feminist positions. For example, in a speech for the American College Health Association, Alan Guttmacher and Gene Vadies criticized the outlook of the handbook produced by students at McGill, which reflected the sensibilities of the nascent women's liberation movement. The authors of the McGill handbook saw birth control as a source of female empowerment rather than containment of world population growth. The McGill students proclaimed their manual was "produced not as a favor to an irresponsible medical profession nor as a favor to men who want an easy but 'safe' lay, but as a political act." They declared that organizations distributing the handbook had a responsibility to ensure that issues of women's liberation were always addressed in discussions of birth control.[53] Guttmacher and Vadies called the McGill handbook "an excellent effort seriously tarnished by mixing leftist political opinions with sex information." As more sensible models, they pointed to "non-political" brochures like *Elephants and Butterflies*.[54] Planned Parenthood also remained adamant that contraception should only be distributed by trained medical professionals and hoped to use student activism to pressure campus health centers to provide reproductive services to students.

These various birth control programs both on and off campus contributed to growing use of the morning-after pill. According to a report in *Medical World News* in 1969, even college physicians who only a few years ago were reluctant to distribute contraceptives to students were now giving postcoital DES to "girls unprepared for the night before." Women were undeterred by the side effects of the morning-after pill. Morris reported that none of his patients failed to complete the course of treatment even if complications were severely uncomfortable. Dr. Douglas McKinnon of the University of California, Los Angeles, concurred, noting that one young woman had to be hospitalized with nausea but nevertheless continued to take the pills.[55]

This rapidly spreading use raised two questions: Was the drug safe? More importantly, was it appropriate for physicians to continue using this technology without filing a new drug application (NDA) with the FDA to seek approval to use DES as a postcoital contraceptive? Celso-Ramon Garcia, at the University of Pennsylvania, stated that when he began their program for rape cases, the hospital's Institutional Review Board asked the FDA whether it needed to file an NDA. The agency said yes, and Garcia's colleague Joseph B. Massey filed an application for postcoital use of DES. Research gynecologists Edward Tyler of Los Angeles and Robert Greenblatt of Augusta, Georgia, said they saw no reason for a new application, arguing that once a drug was approved, other uses could be applied at the discretion of the physician. Dr. Charles Steer, chief of obstetrics and gynecology at Columbia-Presbyterian Medical Center, which oversaw Harlem and Bellevue hospitals, also said an application was not necessary for physicians who wanted to use the drug to prevent pregnancy in rape victims. The FDA conceded that it could not regulate how a physician used a drug already on the market. "Our authority is over the manufacturer and promoter," claimed one official. "We can only advise doctors." The FDA added that the safety and efficacy of DES as a postcoital contraceptive had not been established and that a controlled clinical trial was needed to demonstrate this.[56] The next decade would see further tests of the morning-after pill. Yet, growing criticism of the medical profession's use of human subjects made it less likely that women would continue to serve as courageous volunteers for tests of new contraceptives.

Chapter 3

Feminist Health Activism and the Feds

In October 1971, a University of Michigan Health Service senior physician, Lucile Kirtland Kuchera, published a study of one thousand patients given diethylstilbestrol (DES) as a postcoital contraceptive at the University Health Service in the *Journal of the American Medical Association.* Kuchera had read about the work of Morris and van Wagenen at Yale–New Haven Hospital and began administering their postcoital contraceptive method to patients who came to her for help following unprotected intercourse. Kuchera reported that the pill was 100 percent effective and that no serious side effects were experienced by any of the one thousand women who received the treatment. Some patients reported nausea or headache, but 45 percent had no side reactions.[1] When asked by *New York Times* personal health columnist Jane Brody why she published the study, Kuchera said she wanted not only to confirm the results of other physicians, but also to make general practitioners aware of this treatment.[2]

Physicians and the general public were starting to learn of a more serious consequence of DES: In April of 1971, cancer researchers at Massachusetts General Hospital in Boston published studies that found a high incidence of a rare form of vaginal cancer in the daughters of women who had consumed DES while pregnant.[3] Less than a week after she reported on Kuchera's study, Jane Brody observed in her health column the irony that a national controversy over the cancer-causing properties of DES was brewing at the same time that doctors were proclaiming the effectiveness of the drug as an after-the-fact contraceptive.[4]

The scandal about DES was only the latest in a series of increasingly alarming reports about the failure of the FDA to keep dangerous drugs off the market, especially those marketed to women. By the mid-1960s optimism about the Pill was shaken by reports about blood clots and other serious side effects experienced by some women taking the Pill. *Washington Post* investigative reporter Morton Mintz, who broke the thalidomide story in 1962, also accused the FDA of employing lax standards in approving the contraceptive pill.[5] Starting in the mid-1960s, journalist Barbara Seaman wrote a series of articles about the health risks of hormonal contraception for popular women's magazines such as *Brides* and *Ladies' Home Journal.*

In 1965, the FDA responded to these exposes about the dangers of oral contraceptives by creating the Obstetrics and Gynecology Advisory Committee, the first group of its kind in the agency's history. The advisory committee included physicians and scientists from outside of the FDA, so that the agency could receive independent sources of input. The advisory committee was charged with the task of determining the extent to which oral contraceptives increased the risk of blood clotting, as well as whether the Pill caused cancer of the breast, cervix, or endometrium. The advisory committee seriously considered criticism by Seaman and other consumer activists that the FDA was too easily dismissing women's complaints about the Pill. At their first meeting in November 1965, the committee concluded that it could find no adequate scientific data to justify removing oral contraceptives from the market. Instead, the FDA drew on new regulatory powers granted by the 1962 drug amendments, which not only required drug manufacturers to demonstrate, pre-market, that a new drug was both safe and efficacious, but also gave the FDA the authority to reevaluate the safety and effectiveness of drugs approved prior to 1962. The 1962 amendments also attempted to protect human subjects by requiring investigators to obtain written consent from patients enrolled in experimental drug studies. Finally, manufacturers were required to list contraindications and adverse effects in all drug advertising and had to provide physicians with a package insert to use when advising patients.[6]

These reforms were insufficient for many critics. *Washington Post* columnists Drew Parsons and Jack Anderson accused the FDA of suppressing data in order to protect pharmaceutical companies. In 1969, Seaman published her best-selling exposé, *The Doctors' Case against the Pill,* which roundly condemned scientists, physicians, and the FDA for foisting a dangerous product on unwitting female consumers.[7] In 1970, the Senate Subcommittee on Monopoly of the Select Committee on Small Business, led by Senator

Gaylord Nelson (D-Wisconsin), investigated concerns that the medical profession and the pharmaceutical industry were withholding important information about oral contraceptives from women. No women who had used the birth control pill were called to testify before the Senate subcommittee. The sole female witness was a gynecologist, Dr. Elizabeth Connell, who warned that hyping the dangers of oral contraceptives would cause millions of women to abandon this birth control method and drastically increase the number of unplanned pregnancies in the United States.[8] At the end of the hearings, the FDA commissioner announced the agency would require drug manufacturers to include a patient package insert in every package of birth control pills. The insert had to be written in lay language and include all known side effects and health risks associated with oral contraceptives. The FDA soon caved in to pressure from physicians, who claimed that the insert interfered with the doctor-patient relationship; and manufacturers, who argued that a prescription drug only needed an insert for the physician, not the patient. Feminist groups were angered by the resulting simplified patient insert, arguing that women had a right to full knowledge about the drugs they were taking. These women's health activists also criticized the fact that the hearings excluded testimony from women who had taken the Pill.[9]

Following the Nelson hearings, feminist health activists continued to pressure the federal government to protect women from further abuses by the medical profession. Concerns about the safety of the morning-after pill containing DES became part of this dialogue.

A Burning Issue

The feminist health movement sprang partly from the same self-help impulse that drove the creation of birth control guides on college and university campuses. The feminist health classic, *Our Bodies, Ourselves,* was an extension of the work of college-educated women in the Boston area who set out to gather accurate information about birth control and abortion. They were also interested in other women's health issues such as menstruation, childbirth, gynecological problems, and menopause. However, *Our Bodies, Ourselves* and other feminist health guides differed from other student birth control guides of this era by rooting their activism within the political framework of the women's liberation movement. Unlike liberal feminist groups such as the National Organization for Women (NOW), women's liberation activists believed that it was not enough to fight for laws giving women access to the same educational and job opportunities as men. Instead, the women's liberation movement argued that the main source of women's oppression—male supremacy—had to be dismantled in order for women to achieve full equality. This political perspective was best represented by the demonstrations at the Miss America pageant, organized by New York Radical Women in 1968, during which women liberationists condemned "the Degrading Mindless-Boob-Girlie Symbol" that all women were forced to play.[10]

The group that co-authored *Our Bodies, Ourselves,* the Boston Women's Health Book Collective (BWHBC), emerged from one of the earliest women's liberation conferences in Boston, held at Emmanuel College in 1969. The conference covered a range of women's issues, including the workshop "Women and Their Bodies," at which participants discussed sexuality, abortion, birth control, and childbirth. Everyone who attended this workshop had a story about male doctors who were sexist, paternalistic, or unhelpful. The group continued meeting after the conference, hoping to assemble a list of "good doctors" who would treat women with respect and give them information in a nonjudgmental manner. They soon found that no such physicians existed. The group realized that in order to free themselves from the tyranny of the male-dominated medical profession, they had to find and disseminate knowledge about women's bodies themselves.[11]

Many of these activists argued that while the Pill had freed women from fears of unwanted pregnancy, it had also contributed to male supremacy by increasing pressure on women to submit to the sexual desires of men. One of the authors, Judy Norsigian, recalled that when she was a student at Radcliffe in the late 1960s, and single, "someone sent me to the friendly gynecologist at Harvard Square" for a Pill prescription. The gynecologist told Norsigian, "OK, now we don't have to worry about being pregnant." Yet, access to these helpful yet condescending male doctors willing to prescribe the Pill to unmarried women made it harder for Norsigian and her peers "to say no when we didn't want to have sex" because they could no longer use the excuse "I don't want to get pregnant."[12]

Therefore, the generation of women's health activists who came of age in the 1960s had a different feminist outlook on reproductive rights than did Margaret Sanger. They increasingly criticized the disease-based model of reproductive control that inspired the development of the contraceptive pill. Rather than seeing this technological development aiding women's sexual liberation, they argued that research on the Pill and other compounds used for female reproductive healthcare were part of a larger pattern of mistreatment of women by the medical profession. While these feminists supported Sanger's position on women's rights to bodily autonomy and contraceptive choice, they felt that this goal had been subverted by medical researchers' callous disregard for the safety of their female subjects. These activists also argued that efforts to stem the so-called population crisis disproportionately targeted people of color in the United States and in the developing world.

An example of this new feminist perspective on reproductive rights is the work of Advocates for Medical Information (AMI), a group of female students at the University of Michigan, founded by Belita Cowan, a master's student in Michigan's Department of English. Although this group strongly supported the student health center's decision to offer birth control on campus, they also believed the physicians were exposing young women to excessive health risks in their zeal to protect them from the "disease" of unwanted pregnancy. In 1971, Cowan began an investigation into the use of DES as a morning-after pill at the student health service and the University Medical Center. Cowan worked part-time at the University Medical Center, where physicians routinely gave the drug to female students and other women in the community who wanted to prevent unwanted pregnancies. The student health service advertised this form of contraception in the *Michigan Daily,* the University of Michigan student newspaper. Following a 1969 article in *Medical World News,* health service director Robert E. Anderson confirmed that the drug was being used on the Ann Arbor campus for postcoital contraceptive purposes even though its legality was in doubt. He added that the morning-after pill was also used at the University Medical Center to treat rape victims after doctors there determined the drug was safe for this purpose.[13]

Cowan was horrified that doctors continued to administer DES as a morning-after pill even after the cancer reports began to appear in the medical literature and popular press. She soon organized women who had been patients at the University of Michigan Health Service to form AMI and to protest what they considered to be reckless treatment of women students at the university.[14] Their activism, combined with that of women who had taken DES while pregnant and their daughters, prompted the U.S. House of Representatives Subcommittee of the Committee on Government Operations to begin hearings on DES in November of 1971. At the hearings, FDA commissioner Charles C. Edwards announced that the agency would require manufacturers of DES and related compounds to include a label warning of the association between maternal ingestion of DES during pregnancy and occurrence of vaginal cancer in their daughters. The FDA also mailed a drug information bulletin to all physicians describing the labeling changes and alerting them to search for cancer in young women who might have been exposed in utero. Edwards added that the agency was also considering approving the use of DES as a postcoital contraceptive. He reported that the FDA was reviewing work by Dr. Joseph B. Massey at the University of Pennsylvania, who was conducting a study of the safety and efficacy of DES in preventing pregnancy after alleged rape. To date, Massey had found that only four of five hundred patients in the study had become pregnant and none had exhibited any serious side effects. Edwards had also visited Kuchera at the University of Michigan and was in the process of reviewing the data from her *JAMA* article. He announced that the FDA would continue to study all published data on the subject and meet with drug manufacturers to plan how to obtain scientifically valid information on the safety and efficacy of DES as a postcoital contraceptive. Meanwhile, the FDA would issue a drug bulletin stating that while the use of postcoital DES was widespread, the agency regarded this practice as investigational and could not recommend it without more data to determine the safety and efficacy of this contraceptive method.[15]

A month after the House DES hearings, the FDA Obstetrics and Gynecology Advisory Committee began to consider appeals from physicians to approve including postcoital contraception as one of the indications on the physician package insert for DES. The meetings were led by Dr. Elizabeth Connell, who declared the subject of DES as a postcoital contraceptive was "a burning issue for all of us" in reproductive healthcare. The committee reviewed what they considered to be the scarce clinical data on postcoital contraception, focusing on Kuchera's study, which included the largest patient population up to that point. Dr. H. J. Norris reported on his extensive visit with Kuchera and other University of Michigan health center staff who had cooperated with her study. Norris stated that Kuchera told him that she hoped the committee would approve postcoital use of DES as an indication "because everybody is using it all over the country." Kuchera added that many of the women who came for treatment were so anxious to take the pill they had to be reminded to drink water with it. Dr. Philip Corfman, director of the Center for Population Research, National Institute of Child Health and Human Development (NICHHD), added that other clinicians were hoping the FDA would act quickly on the issue, because they felt uncomfortable administering the drug without FDA approval. The advisory committee discussed the possibility of convincing a pharmaceutical company to file a new drug application for postcoital use of DES. However, Corfman doubted any industry would be willing to invest in such an endeavor because there would be little profit in investigating a product already on the market.[16] More importantly, investigations by feminist groups and consumer advocates would continue to shed a negative light on the morning-after pill.

Coeds as Guinea Pigs

In September 1972, AMI published an article entitled "Cancer and the Morning-After Pill (will you be Mourning-After)" in their feminist newspaper, *her-self*. AMI cofounder Kay Weiss spoke with a participant in Kuchera's study and asked if she had been informed that DES was a powerful carcinogen. The woman replied that the physician had told her the drug was dangerous but not that it could cause cancer. Another woman said she had been told the pills would make her very sick for a few days but nothing about the possible cancer risk of taking DES.[17]

A follow-up article in January 1973 reported that thousands of women took DES during pregnancy and presumably large numbers of female university students had been exposed to DES in utero. Yet no one told these young women they might be at risk for developing vaginal cancer. Instead, many university health services around the country were giving these women more DES in the form of the morning-after pill. Furthermore, even though federal law required that physicians must inform patients of the dangers of a particular drug, doctors continued to tell women that DES was "safe and harmless." The article claimed that women who received the morning-after pill were not given pregnancy tests, nor were they asked if they had a family history of vaginal cancer. When women who had received the drug requested an iodine stain test for vaginal cancer, they were told they were "worrying too much or imaging things because of press reports." This "paternalism," the article argued, usually meant the doctor did not know how to perform the test or had never heard of it.[18]

Members of AIM gave their findings to Dr. Sidney Wolfe and Anita Johnson of Ralph Nader's Health Research Group, who began exploring the use of the morning-after pill on other campuses. In December 1972, Wolfe and Johnson released a report to the Associated Press alleging that many university health centers were prescribing DES as morning-after pills without FDA approval and without informing women of the risk of cancer. The article noted that Dr. Marion Finkel, deputy director of the FDA's Bureau of Drugs, said the agency had been aware for the past year of the widespread use of DES as a morning-after contraceptive and hoped to resolve the issue soon. Finkel added, "We tried to get drug companies interested in doing additional controlled studies but have not been successful," so the agency would need to make a decision without input from manufacturers. The Health Research Group sent a letter to the National Student Association charging that college women were being used as "guinea pigs, without even the most rudimentary observance of professional standards and informed consent."[19] They also sent a letter to University

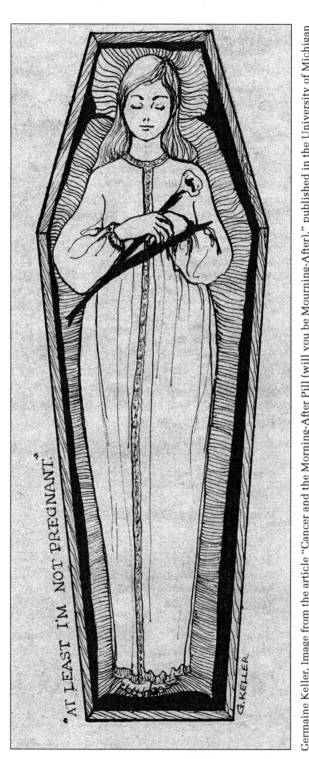

"AT LEAST I'M NOT PREGNANT."

G. KELLER.

Germaine Keller, Image from the article "Cancer and the Morning-After Pill (will you be Mourning-After)," published in the University of Michigan feminist periodical *her-self*, September 1972. Source: Courtesy of the artist and Bentley Historical Library, University of Michigan.

of Michigan president Robben W. Fleming informing him that health service doctors were dispensing DES without informing patients of the risks or doing follow-up on patients to make sure the treatment worked. They acknowledged that while it was admirable that health service doctors wanted to help students desperate to avoid an unwanted pregnancy, DES was an untested method with serious health risks. Johnson and Wolfe strongly urged President Fleming to place controls on use of drugs in the health service and ensure that experiments on students be conducted under the close supervision of a university institutional review board. They concluded, "A great University cannot allow doctors to practice dangerous medicine on its students, however good the intentions all around."[20]

On January 26, 1973, Johnson and Wolfe presented their concerns at a meeting of the FDA Obstetrics and Gynecology Advisory Committee. Wolfe appreciated that the FDA was in a difficult position when it came to drugs that were used off-label, but he was also impatient with claims that the FDA regulated drugs, not doctors, since it left patients vulnerable to health risks from untested medical treatments. Johnson gave a summary of feedback she received from various college and university health centers. She acknowledged that this practice was widespread; and, while a few places followed the recommendations issued by the Health Research Group, most were very careless in how they distributed postcoital contraception. Few issued warnings about the risks of the drug, took medical histories to determine cancer risk, or did much follow-up of patients to determine the outcome of treatment. Two schools—the University of Northern Iowa and the University of Iowa—reported that they did not administer the morning-after pill because of safety concerns. Johnson argued that if the FDA were to allow the use of DES as a morning-after pill, there should be a well-designed study to obtain reliable information and offset risks to human volunteers. Physicians who researched the drug should file an investigational new drug application so that they would be "subject to ongoing surveillance by an institutional review committee" that would ensure that doctors followed procedures of informed consent and did adequate follow-up of the patients. Regardless of whether the FDA approved DES as a morning-after pill, the only way to ensure that DES was used ethically was "to allow the patient to police the use herself" by providing her full information in a patient package insert like those distributed with regular birth control pills. Johnson argued that the history of the morning-after pill indicated that relying on doctors to inform themselves of drug risks was insufficient to protect patients from harm. Instead, drug information should be given directly to the patient so she would not be left out of the decision.[21]

A month later, in February 1973, the issue of postcoital use of DES once again came before Congress, this time at the Senate Subcommittee on Health of the Committee on Labor and Public Welfare hearings on the Quality of Health Care—Human Experimentation. These hearings are best known for exposing the abuse of human subjects in the Tuskegee Syphilis Study.[22] The proceedings also exposed widespread racial and class bias in medical practice regarding women's reproductive health. An entire day was devoted to the high incidence of forced sterilization among poor women of color. The hearings also described female subjects who suffered serious side effects during a trial of the contraceptive Depo-Provera among low-income women attending federally funded family planning clinics.[23]

Extensive discussion of the use of postcoital DES among female college and university students indicated that even privileged women were vulnerable to abusive research practices. The Senate hearings began with FDA commissioner Charles C. Edwards' announcement that the agency was planning to approve postcoital DES for emergency use only. Edwards also summarized the FDA's ability to regulate drugs that had already been approved by the agency. He stated that once a new drug was on the market, physicians could lawfully, as part of the practice of medicine, prescribe the drug for purposes other than that approved in the labeling without first informing or obtaining approval from FDA. Patients had to rely on their doctors to be ethical and reasonably well educated, since FDA could not regulate the practice of medicine. A major difficulty for the FDA was that it was impossible to keep up with the thousands of drug investigations being conducted in the country at any one time. Thus, it was not surprising there were cases where individual investigators like Dr. Kuchera were conducting clinical studies without the agency's oversight. When Senator Edward Kennedy asked who was in a position to oversee these practices, Edwards replied, "I think unfortunately the only recourse today is malpractice." Edwards added, "For too long the medical profession has relied too heavily on the pharmaceutical industry for drug education." Thankfully, most physicians were conscientious and tried to practice good medicine. However, some did not, and there needed to be ways to address this. Senator Nelson agreed that the main concern of the Senate subcommittee was the doctor who relied too heavily on salesmen and advertising in medical journals rather than on scientific articles to get their information on drugs. Edwards stated that the FDA had tried to remedy this by establishing its own publication, the *Drug Bulletin,* to provide physicians with accurate information that was free of drug company marketing. Edwards also proposed that the FDA explore creating a patient package insert for DES, similar to the one already available for oral contraceptives.[24]

The following day, the subcommittee considered whether the limited use of DES as a morning-after pill was justified. The first witnesses were Sidney Wolfe and Anita Johnson, who claimed that the DES morning-after pill was used widely "with unacceptable carelessness, in some cases without even the most elemental requirements of a genuine experiment." At the University of Vermont, follow up was "lackadaisical," and one doctor stated, "We don't dwell on the risks because one-shot use of DES presents no risk to the patient." The University of Oregon health service informed women of the risk of cancer to female offspring and asked them about their family history before the pill was dispensed, but there was no formal follow-up. The Indiana University health service did provide an informed consent form warning of the strong possibility of cancer in offspring and recommending pregnancy termination if DES was ineffective. The consent form also stated that DES had not been approved by FDA for use as a morning-after pill, that the long-term effects of the pill were not known, and that use of well-studied methods of birth control were preferred. This degree of thoroughness was rare, though. At Princeton, women were warned of the cancer risk to offspring but not to themselves. Scripps College, Tufts, Boston University, the University of California–Los Angeles, Syracuse University, the University of Minnesota, Harvard University, Iowa State, and the Feminist Women's Health Center of Los Angeles all dispensed the pill without any cancer warnings. In Washington, the Health Research Group's office manager was able to get a prescription for the pill over the phone with no questions asked and no warnings given. No university health service in the United States had filed an investigational new drug application to use DES as a morning-after pill, and almost none collected data appropriate for such human experimentation. On many campuses there was no uniform policy on what information needed to be given to a woman in order to fulfill conditions of informed consent. Instead, this was "left up to the individual physician" to decide what to tell the patient. One university involved in the study of postcoital contraception had not asked the Institutional Peer Review Committee for their approval: they had simply informed the committee that the research was under way. Johnson argued that students shared the characteristics of guinea pigs and other captive experimental animals in that they were not told what experimenters were doing, nor were they asked if they wanted to participate in research. She also made a direct comparison between the DES studies and the more egregious instances of human subject abuse before the Senate subcommittee. "Whether the subjects are prisoners, college students, military personnel, or poor people, they share a common sense of captivity and the use of drugs on them must be regulated with paramount regard to their well-being," Johnson declared. She and Wolfe called on the senators to institute greater protection of human subjects in experimental settings and suggested that the FDA serve as the central agency for monitoring drug studies in conjunction with university institutional and peer review groups.[25]

In response to the Senate hearings on human experimentation, Congress passed and President Richard Nixon signed the National Research Act (1974), which established the National Commission for the Protection of Human Subjects in Biomedical and Behavioral Research. The act also required formal procedures to protect human subjects, including written consent and institutional review boards to evaluate proposals involving experiments on human beings.[26] Yet, this law had little impact on the use of college and university students as research subjects.[27] This law also did not stop the use of DES as a postcoital contraceptive. In May 1973, an article in the *FDA Drug Bulletin* was mailed to all practicing physicians in the United States, indicating that the FDA had approved postcoital use of diethylstilbestrol (DES), but only as an "emergency measure," not for routine or frequent use as a contraceptive. The bulletin urged physicians to warn patients of possible side effects and advise them of alternative measures available and their hazards so that the patient could make an informed decision about whether to take the drug. Physicians should confirm that the patient was not already pregnant before treatment was administered. If DES therapy failed, the bulletin recommended voluntary pregnancy termination to prevent possible adverse effects on the fetus.[28]

In fact, the FDA had not formally approved the drug; the commissioner had simply received a recommendation to do so from the Obstetrics and Gynecology Advisory Committee. Yet the *Drug Bulletin* announcement gave the implication that the drug had been approved by the FDA for use as a postcoital contraceptive method. Physicians were therefore misled into believing that the FDA had sanctioned use of DES for this purpose. Consequently, this method of contraception became even more widespread, especially at college and university health centers.[29]

This ongoing use of DES would not go unchallenged. Following the Senate hearings on human experimentation in 1973, Cowan conducted her own survey of the morning-after pill, interviewing two hundred women aged eighteen to thirty-one who had taken DES as a postcoital contraceptive in Ann Arbor between 1968 and 1974. She also interviewed nurses, gynecologists, and emergency room doctors at two Ann Arbor hospitals, the University of Michigan Health Service, and several Detroit hospitals. According to the students surveyed, gynecologists at the health center did not tell them about the dangers of DES, nor were they informed that they were part of an experimental study. Contrary to Kuchera's findings, many of those interviewed by Cowan reported extreme side effects. One young woman said, "[I] got so sick from the first pill that I never took the rest. I couldn't stand to be that ill. At the time I took it, the morning-after pill was the new 'fad' on campus, creating an atmosphere in which people were encouraged to be irresponsible in preventive birth control because they thought they could 'take care of it' the next morning. This, unfortunately, did not prove to be as easy or effective as it sounded." Another woman stated, "What still bothers me is the fact that there was such a lack of moral responsibility in dispensing the morning-after pill on an experimental basis without our consent. . . . I feel this incident raises serious questions about the leadership of the Health Service and the ethical standards of many of the doctors who were working there at the time."[30]

At the same time, women who had taken DES during pregnancy and their daughters began a grassroots movement to publicize the dangers of the drug and demand that Congress officially ban its use for any purpose, including postcoital contraception. The founding mother of this movement was Pat Cody, owner of the independent bookstore Cody's Books in Berkeley, who had taken DES while pregnant with her daughter Martha. Cody was already well known in progressive and feminist health circles in the Bay Area: in 1969 she had helped found the Berkeley Free Clinic and, later, its spin-off service for reproductive healthcare, the Berkeley Women's Health Collective. In May 1974, Cody invited the Berkeley health education officer and other healthcare professionals from local clinics and agencies to discuss outreach ideas for DES daughters. Among the twelve women in attendance was Dr. Geraldine Oliva, a pediatrician from the Oakland Children's Hospital Teen Clinic who would later serve as medical director of Planned Parenthood of Alameda County. Oliva and a pediatric oncologist who was an expert in DES gave a demonstration for the staff of the Berkeley Free Clinic on how to examine girls and young women for the signs of vaginal and cervical cancer. Martha Cody served as the DES model and a free clinic staff member served as the non-exposed comparative example. Early in 1975, Cody and other members of what was now called the DES Information Group printed and distributed five hundred copies of a leaflet entitled "Women under 30, Read This," which they distributed to health centers throughout the Bay Area with instructions to duplicate the leaflet for their patients. The DES Information Group also sent each center a fact sheet, clinic procedures, and patient record form for cancer screening that they wrote in conjunction with the Berkeley Women's Health Collective. The Berkeley DES Information Group collaborated with the San Francisco Coalition for the Medical Rights of Women (CMRW), which had started a DES Daughters Committee to spread the word about DES. The CMRW was especially concerned about the continued use of DES as a morning-after pill on college campuses. CMRW reprinted the DES Information Group's leaflet and distributed it to family clinics in San Francisco. Local DES advocacy groups formed around the country and in the mid-1970s came together to form the national organization DES Action.[31] Other feminist health organizations also became involved in DES outreach efforts. The Boston Women's Health Book Collective disseminated information sheets on the drug. These leaflets included warnings about the morning-after pill, stating that the risks of further exposure to DES were uncertain and that the well-informed patient needed to weight the risks and benefits of this treatment carefully.[32]

This activism pressured Congress to raise the subject of DES yet another time, at the Senate Subcommittee on Health hearings on the Regulation of Diethylstilbestrol, held in February 1975. The first statements were made by women who had used DES during pregnancy. When asked by Senator Kennedy what she would say to young women in the United States who were contemplating using the morning-after pill, Mrs. John Malloy of San Diego, California, replied, "Stay away from it, as far away as you can get." Malloy's middle daughter had just graduated from the University of Georgia, where the morning-after pill was handed out indiscriminately even though it was supposed to be used only for emergency purposes. Mrs. Albert Green of Glen Cove, Long Island, a DES mother and acting dean of a school of education in the New York metropolitan area, stated that the young women at her university did not take the morning-after pill just in extreme cases, but often as a regular method of birth control. She was not surprised to learn that the pill was being used just as broadly at other colleges and universities around the country, but added that there should have been more thorough research before the morning-after pill was so widely used.[33]

Dr. Peter Greenwald, director of the Cancer Control Bureau of the New York State Department of Health, stated that although the safety of DES as a morning-after pill had not been proven, its use was fairly widespread, especially at the colleges and universities in New York State. He added that it was used far more broadly than in cases of rape or incest. For most young women, he said, the possibility of an unwanted pregnancy was an emergency, and the morning-after pill was used often in these kinds of situations.[34]

This fact was confirmed by testimony from Cowan, who found that rather than being an emergency medication, DES was being used repeatedly as an ongoing form of contraception. Twenty-nine percent of her sample stated that they had taken the pill at least twice within a one-year period. She also found DES was being prescribed "with carelessness and casualness." Forty-five percent were not given a pelvic exam and 56 percent said the doctor did not take a personal or family medical history. Only 26 percent received follow-up to see if the treatment worked. Rape victims seen in emergency rooms were the least likely to received follow-up care. Most alarming to Cowan was the revelation that DES was being given to women for whom estrogens were contraindicated. Six percent of those surveyed were women who had been exposed to DES in utero. All but one of doctors Cowan interviewed had no reservations about giving the morning-after pill to DES daughters. Sixty-five percent of the women surveyed said that had they been fully informed about DES they would not have taken it. Cowan concluded that "by its failure to regulate the use of DES, the FDA has created a drug abuse problem." Since studies had shown that less than five of every one hundred single, unprotected sexual encounters resulted in pregnancy, she argued, 95 percent of the women receiving DES did not need it. Even rape victims were being exposed unnecessarily to a known carcinogen. Cowan argued that at the very least patients should be informed fully of the risks to themselves and potential offspring. She demanded that there be a patient insert that provided full information on known side effects, contraindications, and alternatives to DES. Physicians should only prescribe DES after taking a thorough medical history, performing a pregnancy test, warning the patient of potential risks, and fully informing her of alternatives such as menstrual extraction and early abortion. Unless these steps were taken, Cowan argued, "DES should not be prescribed to anyone."[35]

Frank Rauscher, director of the National Cancer Institute, said that despite the link between maternal ingestion of DES and cancer in their daughters, women should still have the option of using the drug under limited circumstances and physicians should not be deprived of a useful tool in treating emergency situations. FDA commissioner Alexander Schmidt argued that the agency's decision to approve DES for postcoital contraception was "both justified and in the best interest of the public." This decision, however, came with certain stipulations. Prior to the Senate hearings, the FDA had issued a notice in the *Federal Register* announcing new regulations for drug companies that wished to market DES for postcoital contraception. They also published rules for the content of the patient package insert. Postcoital DES had to be produced in twenty-five milligram tablets and packaged in containers of ten that were available only by prescription. Manufacturers had to provide a patient package insert warning patients of the dangers of DES. The patient insert had to caution that this was to be used as an emergency treatment only and that repeated use should be avoided. Senator Kennedy replied that FDA was putting too much faith in the patient package insert. Senator Richard Schweiker added that even if the package insert was clearly worded, a woman receiving treatment after a rape would be so distraught that the last thing she would do would be to read the insert. She would simply start taking the drug.[36]

Furthermore, these FDA precautions would only be available to consumers if a drug company actually applied and received FDA approval for a product specifically packaged and labeled for use as a postcoital contraceptive. During the Senate hearings, Dr. Robert Furman, vice president of Eli Lilly, the principal manufacturer of DES in the United States, announced the company's decision not to market a twenty-five-milligram dosage form of DES for postcoital contraception. Furman stated that the company had not conducted its own laboratory or clinical investigations to establish the efficacy and safety of DES as a postcoital contraceptive. The company therefore decided to withdraw the line of twenty-five-milligram tablets from the market, and it sent a letter to physicians and pharmacists around the country recommending against using DES for this purpose. Furman added that drug companies had a professional responsibility to conduct their own independent evaluation of the safety and efficacy of a drug before submitting an application to FDA. Senator Kennedy observed that Lilly's decision indicated that the company's standards were actually higher than those developed by FDA in the case of postcoital use of DES.[37]

The only company that chose to apply to the FDA was the New Jersey–based company Tablicaps, a manufacturer of generic drugs. At the Senate hearings on DES, Tablicaps president Robert L. Pillarella testified that his company had submitted an application for a postcoital DES product they called DESMA because the restricted market for this drug was the right size for such a small company and because they believed that rape victims were entitled to the opportunity to have an FDA-approved postcoital contraceptive available. Pillarella argued that rape and incest were growing problems in the United States and that more rapes were being reported because of more humane treatment of victims by police and emergency room personnel. He added that the company would emphasize that DESMA should not be used for routine birth control but for emergency treatment only. He acknowledged that emergency was a difficult thing to define, but argued that physicians should have the discretion to determine what was best for the patient's well-being.[38]

Officials in the FDA Bureau of Drugs were divided on the Tablicaps application. The bureau's director, J. Richard Crout, agreed with the findings of the Obstetrics and Gynecology Advisory Committee that existing scientific studies demonstrated the safety and efficacy of DES as a postcoital contraceptive. The director of the bureau's Generic Drug Division, Dr. Marvin Seife, thought the treatment was too controversial. At the Senate hearings on DES, he added that the publication of postcoital indication for DES in the *Federal Register* was the first time in FDA history that a drug had been promoted by the agency without any investigative new drug application from a pharmaceutical company. Despite pressure from Crout, Seife and his colleagues in the Generic Drugs Division refused to approve Tablicaps' application for DESMA, and the product was never brought to market.[39]

Yet, neither drug manufacturers nor the FDA had control over how physicians chose to use DES in their practices. Despite the controversy raised by the various congressional hearings on the drug, a number of physicians continued to defend using DES for postcoital contraception. William A. Nolen claimed in an article in *McCall's* that the risk of taking DES for five days is "probably negligible." Physicians should not be afraid to use this valuable drug to prevent "the heartache of an unwanted pregnancy."[40] Dr. Celso-Ramon Garcia told *Good Housekeeping* that when compared to the physical and mental consequences of an unwanted pregnancy, DES treatment was much safer. Dr. Arthur Herbst of Massachusetts General Hospital, whose research group first linked DES treatment of pregnant women and cancer in their daughters, said their research only applied to long-term consumption of the drug. They did not have enough evidence from their studies to assess the dangers of DES as a postcoital contraceptive.[41]

The uncertainty about the risks of using DES postcoitally led many birth control providers to either abandon using this contraceptive method or use it sparingly. Although reproductive health experts argued that claims about the dangers of DES as a postcoital contraceptive were based on a very small sample, the concerns about the drug raised by the Senate hearings had succeeded in making everyone—especially those in college health services—cautious about using this method.[42] Planned Parenthood instructed its affiliates not to use DES because their malpractice insurance policy would not cover this treatment. However, the national office did allow affiliates to counsel patients about this contraceptive method, create informational brochures, and refer to other clinics that did offer postcoital treatment.[43] These safety concerns prompted researchers in contraceptive technology and reproductive health professionals to search for an alternative to DES.

Chapter 4

Balancing Safety and Choice

In a 1971 article in *Family Planning Perspectives,* Dr. Philip Corfman, director of the Center for Population Research at the National Institute of Child Health and Human Development (NICHHD), announced the center's five-year plan to fund research to develop new contraceptive methods. The center had been established in August 1968 as part of President Lyndon B. Johnson's administration's efforts to alleviate poverty by providing federal support for contraceptive research and development. Funding for the center continued during the presidency of Richard Nixon, who charged the center to work with other agencies, nonprofit organizations, and the contraceptive industry to develop new birth control methods as rapidly as possible. Corfman observed that the currently available technologies were inadequate to meet the myriad of issues regarding population growth. Many people who used contraceptives—especially teenagers and young adults—failed to use them properly. Others found current methods unacceptable. In particular, recent experience with the contraceptive pill and intrauterine device showed alarmingly high discontinuation rates due to fears about serious health risks and complications. Corfman observed that greater oversight of women using these methods was needed to ensure safe and effective use while scientists continued to develop new contraceptives. Corfman argued that a drug that could be taken only after intercourse had advantages over other methods requiring constant or daily use. In fact, for women who had sex infrequently, a postcoital contraceptive would be ideal because continual medication and its possible side effects would be avoided and the need to remember to take the medication on a regular basis would be unnecessary.[1]

Corfman's description of postcoital contraception as an ideal method for certain users was not new: the first reports on this birth control method framed it as a way to make up for contraceptive "non-compliance," especially among girls and young adults. By the early 1970s, policy makers and population experts were interested in stemming what many considered to be an emerging "epidemic" of unwed teenaged pregnancy in the United States. Like epidemics of other diseases, professionals in public health and reproductive science saw technological innovation as the best way to prevent pregnancy in unmarried teenagers.[2]

The search for a new postcoital contraceptive was also prompted by the outcry from feminist health activists and consumer groups about the safety of DES. In reaction to those protests, the center became interested in finding new drugs that could be substituted for DES. In 1972, the Center for Population Research issued a request for proposals (RFP) for clinical studies of other estrogens as postcoital contraceptive agents.[3]

Contraceptive researchers were not the only ones who were interested in finding a new postcoital contraceptive. Some young women also were eager to use this birth control method. Women read articles about the morning-after pill in the popular press and saw reports about it on major network news broadcasts. While these stories emphasized the safety issues raised by the congressional hearings on DES, they also helped to raise awareness about this contraceptive technology.[4] Workers at rape crisis centers observed that while the use of DES was controversial, some patients asked for it even after they had been warned of possible side effects.[5] Physicians in emergency medicine at the University of New Mexico also found that almost all rape victims they saw "voiced a strong desire to rid themselves of the physical and emotional vestiges of sexual assault."[6] College health professionals reported that they still wrote hundreds of prescriptions for postcoital DES per year. A survey of forty-two health institutions, including the student health services of fourteen large universities and outpatient gynecology services of fourteen major hospitals, conducted by the Cancer Control Bureau of the New York State Health Department indicated that twelve prescribed DES to women directly and eleven others referred them to a physician who would prescribe it. The study estimated that 450 women were treated or referred in New York State alone during 1973, with the heaviest use at college and university health centers.[7] Healthcare professionals at independent abortion clinics also continued to distribute DES to clients who requested it after having unprotected sex.[8] It was this ongoing demand from young women desperate to avoid unwanted pregnancies that played a key role in efforts to find new drugs for postcoital contraception.

Feminist health activists did not necessarily share this enthusiasm for finding a better morning-after pill. In an article in *Ms.* magazine written in response to the RFP, Advocates for Medical Information cofounder Kay Weiss argued that college health centers that agreed to conduct these studies were risking young women's lives in the interest of pursuing lucrative federal contracts. According to Weiss, the money and prestige afforded by federal contracts gave "many institutions ulterior motives." Once again, said Weiss, college coeds all over the country were being entered into experiments without their knowledge or informed consent.[9]

These activists did not ignore the needs of women who had unprotected sex, especially if intercourse was against their will. Rather, they found that the approach of the medical profession was too narrow because it categorized sexual assault as a private tragedy affecting individual women. Instead, these groups increasingly argued that rape was, as New York Radical Feminists put it, "a political crime against women." The first rape crisis centers were started by women from the group DC Women's Liberation who saw the anti-rape movement as an integral part of their larger struggle against oppression of women. The activism of radical feminists eventually compelled the liberal feminist organization the National Organization for Women to enter the arena of anti-rape activism, leading to the creation of the NOW Rape Task Force in 1973.[10]

Although the anti-rape movement, like the women's movement more generally, initially consisted almost entirely of white, middle-class women, it was not long before this branch of feminist action sought ways to bring minority and working-class women into their organizations. According to Washington, D.C., anti-rape activist Loretta Ross, she and other women of color were active in the movement almost from the beginning. Ross was drawn to the anti-rape movement because she had been kidnapped and raped when she was eleven years old and became pregnant at age fourteen in 1968 as a result of incest committed by an older cousin. Legal abortion in the United States was not an option, and her family decided against taking her to Mexico for an abortion because they considered it too dangerous. After delivering her son in a home for unwed mothers, Ross decided to keep the child and give up a scholarship to Radcliffe College. Two years later, Ross became pregnant from a gang rape during her first year at Howard University, but was able to obtain a legal abortion in Washington, D.C. Ross and other women of color were instrumental in convincing white anti-rape activists that racism, poverty, and imperialism were just as important as male supremacy in the struggle to combat violence against women.[11] Eventually, rape became a "bridge issue" that brought together radical, liberal, white women and women of color.[12]

At the same time, women of color pushed for a wider vision of reproductive rights that included a critique of the coercive politics of the mainstream population movement. Women of color resisted externally imposed policies to limit their fertility while asserting their rights to bodily self-determination. For women of color, reproductive freedom meant not only the legal right to abortion and contraception, but also the freedom to have children if they desired.[13]

According to many feminist health activists, the legalization of abortion in 1973 gave rape victims a safer option for preventing pregnancy than the morning-after pill. In addition, feminist groups, such as the Jane collective in Chicago, that had offered reproductive health services prior to legalization of abortion remained critical of the medical model of abortion that narrowly focused on treating the "disease" of unwanted pregnancy rather than the larger issue of women's reproductive self-determination. Instead, groups like Jane were based on a feminist political perspective that used abortion services as an entry point to raise women's consciousness about their rights to control their own bodies. These groups insisted that feminist health activism did not end with making abortion safe and legal, but needed to ensure the woman-centered principles remained paramount in the post-*Roe* era.[14] This ongoing insistence on feminist self-determination in healthcare and vigilance toward drug safety would continue to shape the feminist health community's response to research on postcoital contraceptives during the 1970s and 1980s.

Searching for Specific Scientific Data

The NIH-funded studies were an attempt to make sense of years of ad hoc use of postcoital contraception in the United States. Richard P. Blye, a pharmacologist from the center's Contraceptive Development Branch, observed that use of postcoital contraception had expanded rapidly since John McLean Morris and Gertrude van Wagenen's work was published in the mid 1960s. News about the postcoital pill was spread among physicians through the medical literature and to young women through self-help guides produced at colleges and universities during the late 1960s and early 1970s.[15] Renee Chelian recalled that when she first graduated from high school, she worked for a gynecologist in Detroit, Michigan, who began offering "morning-after treatment" in the late 1960s. She soon spread word about this contraceptive method to her friends and former high school classmates.[16] Claire Keyes, executive director of Allegheny Reproductive Health Center in Pittsburgh, Pennsylvania, remembers that the two African American physicians who worked at the center, Dr. Robert L. Thompson and Dr. Robert Kisner, were early pioneers in providing postcoital contraceptive pills to patients in the Pittsburgh area.[17] By the early 1970s, the technology was widespread, especially on college campuses. However, Blye and other scientists at NIH observed that there was little specific scientific data documenting use of estrogens for this purpose.

In order to assess clinicians' experiences with postcoital contraception, the Center for Population Research held a working session on the topic at the NIH on February 14, 1972. Participants included FDA Obstetrics and Gynecology Advisory Committee members, representations from the Population Council and Planned Parenthood, and a number of physicians who were using postcoital contraception in emergency rooms at urban hospitals and in student health centers. The majority of attendees at the workshop used DES as the postcoital contraceptive agent. Corfman began the meeting by explaining that the FDA Obstetrics and Gynecology advisory committee was uncertain about the safety and efficacy of DES for pregnancy prevention following unprotected intercourse. The advisory committee wanted further evidence from clinicians who were currently using the drug as a postcoital contraceptive. Corfman also announced that NIH would like to explore the use of other estrogens for this purpose. Dr. Edwin M. Ortiz, director of the FDA Division of Metabolic Drug Products, pointed out that while the American College of Obstetrics and Gynecology had recognized DES as a standard treatment for rape victims, it was not so designated on the drug's physician package insert approved by the FDA. He also mentioned that he had approached several drug companies with the suggestion of doing clinical trails, but none were interested in funding any further research on this topic. Morris presented his earlier work on DES and further studies he had conducted with van Wagenen on ethinyl estradiol.[18] Lucille Kuchera provided an update on her work with DES.[19] Takey Crist reported on his study of the conjugated estrogen product Premarin as a postcoital contraceptive at the Obstetrics and Gynecology Department of North Carolina Memorial Hospital. Of the 194 women who sought postcoital treatment, none became pregnant. Seventeen percent experienced nausea, dizziness, or vomiting, but these symptoms were not severe enough to discontinue treatment. Crist also provided results of his survey of North Carolina physicians regarding use of postcoital contraception. Only 30 percent of the 3,800 physicians Crist contacted replied to the survey. Of those, 82.5 percent said they did not use postcoital contraception or did not know of the treatment, and 17.5 percent said they had prescribed or offered the drug. The most common agent used was DES but some used Premarin or Depo Provera.[20]

Dr. Hans Lehfeldt, a private practitioner in New York City, presented his work on ethinyl estradiol as a postcoital contraceptive. Of the 105 patients he treated, only 1 became pregnant, and that patient had been treated nine days after unprotected intercourse. Lehfeldt also gave results of a much larger study of ethinyl estradiol conducted by Dutch researcher Ary Haspels in the Netherlands. Haspels first used the compound as a resident in obstetrics and gynecology in Amsterdam. In 1964, the Amsterdam police brought a thirteen-year-old rape victim to the ob-gyn department. Haspels and the other residents consulted with a veterinarian about the use of estrogen in canines following "unwanted mating." They administered the drug to the girl and prevented the pregnancy. Haspels then continued to use ethinyl estradiol as a postcoital contraceptive; and after Morris and van Wagenen's work on DES appeared in 1966, Haspels used that drug as well. In 1972, Haspels published the results of treatment of two thousand women aged fourteen to fifty-two years. There were a total of fourteen pregnancies in this series, four among those administered DES, and ten using ethinyl estradiol.[21]

Dr. George Langmyhr from Planned Parenthood–World Population presented the results of a poll he conducted of the organization's affiliates. He found that use of DES as a postcoital contraceptive was highly successful in preventing pregnancy. Yet he also mentioned that many of the clinics were afraid to use the technique because of liability concerns. Planned Parenthood wanted guidelines from FDA as well as funds for research and follow-up studies. Dr. Elizabeth Connell reported on a study she had conducted among clinicians in New York State. She stated that she had sent questionnaires to various hospitals and colleges in New York State, finding that "there is a lot of use, but nobody knows what they are doing." Many used the treatment randomly, with little to any follow-up in most cases. Dr. Celso-Ramon Garcia gave the results of his and Joe B. Massey's work on rape victims treated at the University of Pennsylvania. There were four pregnancies among the 186 women treated. Garcia added that the study of this group of patients was difficult as it was hard to do adequate follow-up.[22]

In March 1972, Corfman's colleague at NIH, Daniel Seigel, summarized the results of the workshop to the FDA Obstetrics and Gynecology Advisory Committee. Seigel found that the drugs were used mainly in three settings—student health centers, family planning clinics, and city hospitals—and that the most accessible data on efficacy came from colleges and universities, which had the best follow-up of their patient populations. The general consensus of the workshop was that a cooperative study with a standardized protocol was necessary to establish the legitimacy of DES and other estrogens for postcoital contraception. Seigel announced that the NICHHD should be the one to file a new drug application for postcoital estrogens with FDA since the private sector was unlikely to do so because there was no profit in it. This proposal was highly unusual, since applications for approval of new drugs typically came from manufacturers, not from medical experts outside of the pharmaceutical industry.[23]

Within a few years of the release of the first RFP for studies of postcoital estrogens, the NICCHD had awarded grants to Planned Parenthood clinics in Connecticut and Minnesota and student health centers affiliated with Baylor Medical School, the University of Pittsburgh, and the University of Florida to test the efficacy and safety of estrogens that could be substituted for DES as postcoital contraceptives. By 1977, the five study centers had enrolled a total of 1,311 women seeking postcoital contraceptive treatment. One of the centers used conjugated estrogens, two used ethinyl estradiol, and two alternated between the two drugs.[24]

In order to be enrolled in the study, women had to be between the ages of eighteen and thirty-five, have only one unprotected act of intercourse in the middle of their menstrual cycle, and have no contraindications for use of estrogens, such as a history of cancer of the reproductive tract, breast, or pituitary. Study subjects could not have used postcoital contraception in the past, nor could they currently be using oral contraceptives. All eligible women were required to provide written, informed consent and a full record of their menstrual histories. They received full physical and gynecological exams and pregnancy tests prior to receiving treatment. Subjects also had to abstain from intercourse during the treatment cycle, keep a record of side effects and onset of menses, and return to the clinic for follow-up exams and pregnancy tests within thirty to sixty days after their initial visit.[25]

Of the 1,311 women originally enrolled in these clinical studies, the research centers were able to complete case histories on all but 47 women who did not return for follow-up care. Of the remaining 1,264 women who completed the full study protocols, 12 became pregnant, a rate of less than 1 percent. The studies also demonstrated that ethinyl estradiol was slightly more effective in preventing pregnancy, as women who received this compound were less likely to conceive than those receiving conjugated estrogens. Postcoital estrogen therapy also was more effective if given within twenty-four hours of unprotected intercourse.[26]

In an article on their study at the University of Florida, Morris Notelovitz and David Sayre Bard summed up the implications of their research: "There is a large group of sexually active young women who are reluctant to seek contraceptive advice and protection until after the fact." Some women hesitated to obtain birth control because of embarrassment. Others could not afford contraceptives and/or doctors' visits. Some women felt that oral contraceptives and intrauterine devices were "indicative of implied permissiveness" or caused severe complications. A number of women, though, were exposed to unprotected intercourse due to rape or method failure such as broken condoms or displaced diaphragm or IUD.[27] Thus, it was clear to these researchers that there was a need for an effective back-up method of contraception. Balancing the search for a new method of postcoital contraception with the safety concerns of consumer activists would prove to be a challenge.

The Voice of the Women's Health Movement on Capitol Hill

On December 15, 1975, a group of Washington, D.C., area women's health activists held a memorial service on the steps of the FDA building to commemorate the thousands of women who died because of complications from the contraceptive pill, DES, and hormone replacement therapy. The service was the public face of the group's participation in the various congressional hearings on DES and other estrogens. The day after the memorial service, Belita Cowan and several other members of this group testified at the House hearings on the use of DES as a morning-after pill. The public demonstration and congressional testimony grew out of the efforts of Cowan and other feminist health activists—including Barbara Seaman, Phyllis Chesler, Mary Howell, and Alice Wolfson—to enhance the lobbying efforts of feminist health activists in the nation's capital. In May of 1976, the group organized a national conference of other women activists from around the country. At the conference attendees elected a twelve-member board of directors for a National Women's Health Network (NWHN) to serve as a watchdog of FDA and other federal health agencies and ensure that the voice of the women's health movement was heard on Capitol Hill.[28]

The creation of the NWHN represented the growing professionalization of the women's health movement in the United States. Feminist health activists realized that in order to enhance their efficacy as advocates for women health issues, they needed to become political insiders: this included earning the professional credentials and gaining the scientific knowledge necessary to speak the language of other experts who testified on the safety and efficacy of various contraceptive methods during the 1970s and 1980s.[29]

This professional approach was already evident in feminist health activists' testimony at the DES hearings, where Cowan presented data from her own survey of women who had used the morning-after pill. As the NWHN gained experience on Capitol Hill, members became increasingly adept at using the same standards of scientific evidence as other expert witnesses. This ability to use the same terms as the medical establishment is exemplified by the testimony of NWHN board member Judy Norsigian before the House Select Committee on Population in 1978. The hearing was organized to weigh evidence questioning the safety of various contraceptive methods being explored by federally funded population research, nonprofit organizations such as the Population Council and Planned Parenthood, and drug companies. Norsigian stated that "those of us active in the women's health movement are concerned that present funding is too heavily weighted toward drug and device research" and that "too often, such research has exposed human subjects, mostly women, to serious adverse consequences." Norsigian referred to hundreds of "nightmare stories" sent to her and the other editors of *Our Bodies, Ourselves* describing the serious side effects women had suffered from the Pill, Depo Provera, and the Dalkon Shield intrauterine device. Norsigian observed that most contraceptive researchers were male and hence had "little direct understanding of the practical impact of their research on women." Norsigian said that male bias was evident in the policy recommendations on federal population research, which gave priority almost exclusively to drugs and devices meant for women. "We doubt if a committee composed primarily of women—consumers as well as researchers and government administrators—would have presented a similar list of recommendations."[30]

As an alternative to potentially dangerous drugs and devices, Norsigian and other NWHN members endorsed the self-help model developed by feminist women's health centers in the 1960s and 1970s. Norsigian argued that the medical profession had emphasized the "presumed passivity of women" and placed too much faith in contraceptive methods requiring little or no active participation from users. This attitude was especially apparent in the case of teenagers and young women. In the zeal to do anything to prevent the "epidemic" of unplanned teenage pregnancies, Norsigian said, population experts had too easily disregarded issues of safety. Norsigian argued that safety considerations were especially important when addressing the contraceptive needs of adolescent girls. Because the long-term affects of oral contraceptives on female reproductive development were unknown, prescribing hormonal contraception to adolescents was unwise. Norsigian argued that based on her work with inner-city youth in the Boston area, the self-help model used in many women's health centers improved effective use of barrier methods and the ovulation method, even among teenage women. Yet, these safer birth control methods did not receive priority from granting agencies, while potentially dangerous methods attracted the majority of funds.[31]

The position of the NWHN was that "women should be creating policy on behalf of women" and "at the very least, that all users of contraceptives should have a significant voice in determining what kind of research is funded." In particular, there needed to be more research conducted by community-based women's health centers that worked directly with those who would benefit the most from this research. As a model for this women-centered research, the NWHN conducted a survey of over one hundred women's health centers and women's health education groups to determine what these organizations saw as their contraceptive research priorities.[32] The NWHN would also continue to play a role in evaluating new postcoital contraceptive methods that were reviewed by the FDA.

A Catch-22 for the FDA

At the April 11, 1980, meeting of the FDA Fertility and Maternal Health Drugs Advisory Committee (formerly the Obstetrics and Gynecology Advisory Committee), Richard Blye and Dr. Howard Ory, chief of Family Planning Evaluation Branch of the Centers for Disease Control, presented an overview of the studies of postcoital contraception funded by the Center for Population Research. The committee was chaired by David F. Archer, who had conducted the study of postcoital estrogens at the University of Pittsburgh. Philip Corfman commended the FDA for its willingness to take on a topic of considerable significance to the public health without first being prompted to do so by drug manufacturers. In the case of DES, the FDA Obstetrics and Gynecology Advisory Committee had provided some guidance to physicians on proper use of this drug as a method of preventing pregnancy. Corfman hoped the advisory committee would do the same with other estrogens used as postcoital contraceptives.[33]

The advisory committee also heard testimony from Belita Cowan, who appeared on behalf of the NWHN. Like other consumer groups during the 1970s, the NWHN demanded and received a greater role in determining the safety and efficacy of new drugs and devices. The Freedom of Information Act gave consumer activists and other private citizens greater access to deliberations that had formerly been restricted to federal officials and industry insiders. These activists not only were interested in receiving information, but also insisted they had a right to influence decisions about what products came to and remained on the market. In response to these demands, the FDA under the direction of Charles Edwards expanded its advisory committee structure and permitted testimony from consumer rights groups like NWHN.[34]

Cowan claimed that the data on safety and efficacy presented by Blye and Ory was insufficient to justify a recommendation that FDA approve ethinyl estradiol and conjugated estrogens as postcoital contraceptives. As in the case of DES, Cowan's chief concern was the possibility of fetal exposure should treatment fail. She further stated that fetal exposure to high doses of estrogens had been linked to cardiovascular and limb reduction defects. Therefore, follow-up for fetal exposure was essential for postcoital pill users. She asked whether prescribing doctors would provide abortion services if the postcoital pill did not work, and if physicians would be held liable should the injured offspring come of age and attempt to bring lawsuits. In addition, Cowan argued that the possibility of risk to users themselves was significant. In her investigation of Kuchera's work at the University of Michigan, Cowan found that DES daughters had been given postcoital DES. Other women in the study, who were not DES daughters, relied on the postcoital pill as an occasional, and sometimes frequent, method of contraception. Although the risk of postcoital estrogens was unknown, there were known risks such as cancer and cardiovascular problems associated with other estrogen drugs. Cowan and other members of NWHN concluded that the sample size provided by the NIH studies was too small to justify a move toward FDA approval for postcoital estrogens.

Archer observed that one of the things physicians could offer a young woman was reassurance that she would not get pregnant. He asked Cowan what alternative methods the NWHN would suggest. Cowan replied that until the safety of postcoital estrogens was determined and the efficacy confirmed, she suggested that physicians wait to see if menses returned spontaneously. If the woman's period was late, she recommended using the self-help technique of menstrual extraction developed by women's health clinics and consciousness-raising groups as a way for women to regulate their bodies independently of the medical establishment. The procedure involved using plastic cannula and mild suction to remove the uterine lining on or about the first day of an expected menstrual period. Although menstrual extraction was used mostly to relieve the pain and inconvenience of menstruation, women's health groups and some independent abortion providers also used the procedure in cases when a woman's menstrual period was late and/or she feared she was pregnant because of unprotected intercourse.[35] Cowan concluded, "I think it is always prudent to be cautious, and if we can spare people from unnecessary medication, I think we should go in that direction."[36]

Blye replied that most medical experts and the federal government considered menstrual extraction to be equivalent to abortion. Advisory committee
member William Easterling added that menstrual extraction "can be a very
traumatic experience for a woman" and that his institution had stopped
offering the procedure. William Andrews agreed that menstrual extraction
was not the safest alternative because the failure rate was significant. He argued
that taking postcoital contraception was less stressful for a woman than having
to go through the trauma of an abortion.[37]

Phyllis Wetherill, head of the DES Registry, stated that she was concerned
that college campuses were already leading patients to believe that these
other estrogens were safer than DES without any firm evidence that this was
true. She agreed that women wanted choice, especially in a crisis situation,
so she did not want to get rid of the postcoital pill entirely. She called on the
committee to exert whatever effort it could to issue a letter to physicians and
a patient package insert warning of the risks of postcoital estrogens to women
who had already been exposed to DES.[38]

Corfman claimed that the availability of a postcoital contraceptive simply
expanded "the freedom of women to control their own reproductive functions."
He proposed that FDA require that the patient insert for oral contraceptive pills
and other estrogen drugs used for hormone replacement include a special
section on postcoital contraception for the patient to read. Women would be
instructed that this treatment was for emergency use only, that they should not
repeat the medication, and that if they should become pregnant should have
an abortion. As in the case of DES, Corfman said, it would be better for public
policy for FDA "to take a position on the appropriate use of this medication,
rather than to let it just ride freely."[39]

Archer replied that the FDA faced a "bureaucratic Catch-22": unless a
company filed a new drug application to use ethinyl estradiol or conjugated
estrogens as postcoital contraceptives, with specific labeling for that use,
then the FDA could not put information about postcoital contraception in
the patient package insert for these drugs. All they could do was encourage
industry to file a new drug application and publish information for physicians
in the FDA *Drug Bulletin*. Bernard H. St. Raymond, fertility and infertility
division leader of the FDA's metabolism branch, warned that even a notice in
the FDA *Drug Bulletin* would imply that the agency had officially approved
estrogens for postcoital use.[40]

Because of the safety issues and lawsuits that arose from the DES scandal,
drug companies were not interested in filing applications for postcoital use of

ethinyl estradiol or conjugated estrogens. In an article on the FDA advisory committee meeting in *Medical World News,* a spokesman from Ayerst said the company had no plans to change the label for Premarin, a conjugated estrogen used for hormone replacement therapy, to include postcoital contraception as an indication for the drug.[41] This did not stop professionals in reproductive health from continuing to search for something to help their patients avoid unwanted pregnancy.

The Yuzpe Method

At the same time as the NICCHD studies were under way in the United States, researchers in Canada were looking for a safer alternative to DES. Like their counterparts in the United States, students at Canadian colleges and universities demanded access and received to birth control services during the 1960s and 1970s.[42] Access to abortion was more restricted in Canada than the United States. Although the Canadian government legalized abortion in 1969, a woman could receive an abortion only if her life or health were in danger. Under Canadian law, hospital therapeutic abortion committees were needed to approve an abortion, but only a small percentage of Canadian hospitals established such committees and most of these were in large urban areas. Women frequently had to travel long distances within or outside of Canada to obtain an abortion. This situation made finding a safe and reliable method of postcoital contraception even more urgent in Canada than in the United States.[43]

To respond to these kinds of reproductive health needs, associate professor of obstetrics and gynecology A. Albert Yuzpe began a gynecology clinic at the University of Western Ontario Student Health Service in 1970. The university president at the time, D. Carlton Williams, was concerned with the growing rate of unwed pregnancy at the university and believed that providing contraceptives in the student health service would help alleviate this problem. Despite the availability of birth control on campus, Yuzpe found that 60 percent of the women he saw in the clinic had not used contraceptives during their first act of sexual intercourse, and 40 percent were unprotected or inadequately protected during subsequent sexual experiences. As in the United States, Canadian physicians were increasingly reluctant to use DES as a postcoital contraceptive due to concerns about the link between the drug and cancer. Yuzpe was aware of Haspels's work on ethinyl estradiol in the Netherlands. He also knew that researchers in Hong Kong had used the progestin compound levonorgestral as a postcoital contraceptive and found that women had fewer side effects such as nausea and vomiting than they did with estrogen compounds. In Canada, the only pharmaceutical product on the market that contained levonorgestral was the combination oral contraceptive Ovral, which contained both the progestin compound and ethinyl estradiol.[44]

During the 1972–73 academic year, Yuzpe launched a pilot study of Ovral as a postcoital contraceptive, treating a total of 143 women aged eighteen to forty-two years. The researchers used the student newspaper and other methods of campus publicity to solicit volunteers for their study. Their results were comparable to those obtained using DES, but there were considerable advantages to using Ovral: first, the pills were administered as a single dose, while DES had to be taken in fifty milligram doses per day for a five-day period. More importantly, because Ovral was a commonly used oral contraceptive, the "certain degree of fear" that women had about DES was eliminated. Yuzpe realized that the study sample at the University of Western Ontario was small, and several years later he extended his work to include four additional university health services in Canada. In this study, Yuzpe and his colleagues chose to implement a new dosage of two Ovral tablets followed by two tablets twelve hours later. Of the 464 patients enrolled in this larger study, only one became pregnant. Once again, Yuzpe emphasized the importance of these findings in addressing the problem of unwed pregnancy in university women, as well as the growing number of pregnancies resulting from sexual assault.[45]

In the United States, Yuzpe's findings were duplicated by Dr. Lee H. Schilling, staff gynecologist at the California State University, Fresno, student health service. The study, conducted during the spring 1978 semester, enrolled 115 students, none of whom became pregnant. Schilling observed that despite the growing use of other estrogens for postcoital contraception, to many, DES and the morning-after pill were synonymous. The link between DES and cancer had "created confusion" not only about the safety of DES but that of postcoital contraception more generally. As a result of "perceived dangers" about the use of estrogens, postcoital contraception was "a poorly understood and vastly underutilized tool."[46]

In 1980, *Contraceptive Technology Update,* a newsletter for professionals in reproductive healthcare, published a report on Yuzpe's and Schilling's findings. The article described the ease of the Ovral method: clinicians could simply punch out four tablets from a regular package of the oral contraceptive and give them to the patient while she was in the office. Instructions for how to take Ovral—two tablets immediately, the other two twelve hours later—were easier to explain to the patient than the five-day regimen for DES. Patients were also less likely to experience nausea and vomiting while taking Ovral and were thus more likely to complete the course of treatment. Most importantly, women and practitioners who were hesitant to use DES might feel more comfortable using Ovral. Both Yuzpe and Schilling found that measured against the risks of pregnancy and abortion, the danger of using Ovral as a postcoital contraceptive was lower since it entailed fewer medical complications and avoided the financial, social, and psychological costs of abortion.[47]

Contraceptive Technology Update's editor, Robert A. Hatcher, professor of gynecology and obstetrics at the Emory University School of Medicine, confirmed these findings. Hatcher had adopted Yuzpe's method as a rape treatment protocol at Grady Memorial Hospital in Atlanta. Hatcher's work also demonstrates the impact that the contraceptive self-help movement among college students in the 1960s was beginning to have on the medical profession. In 1972, Hatcher collaborated with James Trussell on a popular advice book, *Women in Need.* This book incorporated the same scathing critique of racial and class prejudice within the population movement that Trussell had made in *The Loving Book.* According to Trussell and Hatcher, "the contention that the poor do not want to limit their family size is highly suspect." This claim was made by those who subscribed to the "culture of poverty" hypothesis posed by Oscar Lewis, who alleged that persons living in poverty are "fatalistic, have a low level of aspiration, and generally do not plan." Drawing on the work of Steve Polgar and Frederick Jaffe, Trussell and Hatcher called this hypothesis a "cop-out." They argued that the real obstacle to family planning was "the perception of the establishment rather than the life-style of the poor." It was no wonder that black militants viewed family planning programs as a white plot aimed at reducing the welfare rolls rather than empowering women of color to control their own reproductive lives. In order to be successful, family planning programs had to emphasize the view that birth control is "an aid to enable women, all women, to have children when they want to." Furthermore, if family planning programs were not accompanied by other programs to improve the material lives of the poor—better housing, better education, better jobs, and better access to quality healthcare in general—"—"then the charges of the black minority who now oppose birth control will ring more true to the entire black community."[48]

This increasingly progressive view of reproductive health was also exemplified by the work of another one of Hatcher's colleagues, Felicia Hance Stewart. Stewart's background illustrates how second-wave feminist health activism influenced female physicians who entered the field of women's reproductive health during the 1960s and 1970s. Stewart pursued her undergraduate degree at the University of California, Berkeley, and received her MD from Harvard during the heyday of student activism in the 1960s. Her commitment to advancing women's reproductive rights was confirmed during her internship in the early 1970s when she witnessed the death of a young woman who had suffered an unsafe abortion. Following her residency at the University of California, San Francisco, she and her husband started a fertility clinic and obstetrics and gynecology practice in the Bay Area that incorporated many of the principles of woman-centered healthcare and demedicalized childbirth that were promoted by feminist health activists. The couple also worked on behalf of nurse midwives and led a successful lobbying effort in California to allow these practitioners to deliver babies and perform abortions. Her advice manual for patients, *My Body, My Health* (1979), adopted the model of female empowerment through bodily self-knowledge promoted by *Our Bodies, Ourselves* and other feminist health books. She was among a number of gynecologists who taught other healthcare professionals about the Yuzpe method. Stewart collaborated with Hatcher and other physicians to get that description of this technology included in articles and textbooks for professionals in women's reproductive health.[49]

In an editorial in *Contraceptive Technology Update* in 1980, Hatcher declared that postcoital contraception could not only prevent unwanted pregnancy but also "unlock the healthcare door" for women who did not realize they needed regular reproductive healthcare or family planning. These women included not only rape victims, but teenagers, college students, and separated, divorced, or widowed women who had sex infrequently. According to Hatcher, with postcoital contraception, reproductive health professionals could do more than offer help in a crisis situation, they could also reintroduce women to the health-care delivery system and thereby extend "a greater awareness of [women's] own health."[50]

The Ovral regime, nicknamed the Yuzpe method after the Canadian physician's pioneering work in this area, was approved by drug regulatory agencies in Great Britain and West Germany in the early 1980s. Yuzpe hoped that the same would happen in the United States and Canada.[51] Yet pharmaceutical companies were unwilling to apply to either the U.S. Food and Drug

Administration or the Canadian Marketed Health Products Directorate to have oral contraceptives relabeled for postcoital contraception. In an article in *Contraceptive Technology Update* entitled "Postcoital Contraception: A Delicate Political Issue," Wyeth marketing representative for Canada Gurt Jurgneit said that the company was not enthusiastic about marketing such a method. For years, the company had been telling women not to take oral contraceptives if they were pregnant. The postcoital regimen entailed telling women to take a higher dose of Ovral if they suspected they might become pregnant. Explaining the difference between the two uses of Ovral would be a problem, he said.[52] Wyeth's manager of public relations in the United States, Audrey Ashby, stated that the company did not advise practitioners to use Ovral as postcoital contraception and would not support health providers who gave this contraceptive method to their patients and later encountered legal problems.[53]

The lack of FDA approval for the Yuzpe method made it difficult for healthcare providers to learn about this technology because this information was not available on the package insert for oral contraceptive pills nor was it readily available in most medical or nursing textbooks. A survey conducted by *Contraceptive Technology Update* in the mid-1980s indicated that the majority of respondents did not offer postcoital contraception to their patients largely because they were unaware of the method. Three-fourths of all nurse practitioners and nurse midwives had never prescribed postcoital pills, while only slightly more than half of all physicians had done so. Furthermore, liability concerns made it impossible for some providers to administer the Yuzpe method to their patients. Federally funded family planning services could not prescribe or distribute drug regimens that did not have FDA approval.[54] Planned Parenthood's insurer would not cover them for postcoital contraception. Eve Paul, director of Legal Services for Planned Parenthood, instructed affiliates to refer patients seeking this birth control option to outside agencies.[55] Independent abortion clinics tended not face the same restrictions as did Planned Parenthood clinics and became one of the most common places outside of emergency rooms and student health services where women could obtain the Yuzpe method.[56]

Thus, despite two decades of research on postcoital contraception, this technology remained unknown to many health professionals and most of the general public. At the same time, feminist health activists continued to raise concerns about the safety of postcoital contraception and the potential mistreatment of female research subjects through ongoing research on this contraceptive method. For these activists, abortion and the self-help technique of menstrual extraction were better back-up methods of contraception because they did not involve using drugs that had not been demonstrated conclusively as safe and effective. This perspective was made possible because of recent advances in women's access to contraception and abortion. The erosion of these reproductive rights, especially for minors and low-income women, during the ensuring decade would prompt the women's health movement to reevaluate their position on postcoital contraception.

Chapter 5

Building Consensus

In June of 1979, a group of healthcare professionals, scientists, lay midwives, consumer advocates, social scientists, women's studies professors, historians, and policy analysts held a workshop entitled "Ethical Issues in Human Reproduction Technology: Analysis by Women" at Hampshire College in Amherst, Massachusetts. This workshop was the first conference in the United States to focus on women's views of the ethical issues of reproductive technology. Topics included hormonal contraception, sterilization abuse, diethylstilbestrol and cancer, prenatal diagnosis, neonatology, and assistive reproductive technologies such as in vitro fertilization and embryo transfer. The conference participants challenged two key assumptions of contraceptive research and development: first, that the "disease" of unwanted pregnancy was worse than the health risks posed by a contraceptive technology; and, second, that the threat of overpopulation was a greater social problem than the health and welfare of women living in poverty. Although participants supported offering women a diverse range of choices of contraceptive methods, they also favored noninvasive methods that posed the least risk of long-term side effects. In particular, they recognized that a safe back-up method of contraception was needed for rape victims and for cases where other contraceptive methods failed. Belita Cowan presented her work on the ethical issues of research on postcoital contraceptives. She pointed out that until recently the various federal agencies that oversaw contraceptive research were staffed almost entirely by white males. Thus, key decisions about which studies to fund and which technologies to approve were made by those who would never have to face the health risks posed by the various drugs and devices created for fertility control. Cowan claimed that this led to serious ethical lapses in contraceptive research: in the case of studies of postcoital contraception, it was unclear whether the women were aware they were part of an experiment or if they knew they were taking a drugs that the FDA had never approved for this use. Cowan concluded that women "have come to learn, in a very painful way, that men think of us as statistics, that their risk/benefit ratios often ignore our health needs and our concern for safety as well as efficacy." Because birth control was still primarily women's responsibility and women bore the consequences of pregnancy and childbirth as well as the health risks posed by various contraceptive technologies, "women should have the major voice in determining which contraceptive research priorities best meet our needs."[1]

Helen Holmes observed that while feminist health activists favored contraceptive methods with little chance of long-term side effects, a safe, nontraumatic method of postcoital contraception was needed in case of failure of other techniques and in case of rape. However, she stated, "most postcoital methods are risky and future technological solutions may well be also." Therefore, she concluded, "confronting the context of rape becomes an issue in contraceptive technology."[2]

Feminist health activists were not the first to consider postcoital contraception in the context of rape: the earliest use of this birth control method was for the treatment of victims of sexual assault. However, feminist involvement in combating the problem of rape extended beyond medical solutions that only addressed preventing unwanted pregnancy. Instead, feminist activists in the anti-rape movement saw sexual assault as part a larger systemic pattern of male dominance in American culture. Likewise, Holmes suggested that considering rape and contraceptive technology from a feminist perspective involved more than developing a new postcoital contraceptive method. Rather, educating about rape, setting up rape crisis centers, caring for battered women, stopping pornography, and curbing violence against women were all issues that needed to be considered in the context of reproductive technology. In terms of ways to prevent pregnancy in rape victims, she and many others at the conference favored the feminist self-help procedure of menstrual extraction.[3]

Participants at the Ethical Issues workshop were not united on the issue of postcoital contraceptive pills. In her response to Cowan's presentation, sociologist Kristin Luker stated that the central question was one of choice, which included not only providing a range of options, but also allowing women to make their own decisions about whether the benefits of a contraceptive technology outweighed the potential risks. Luker noted that she had spent the 1970s telling officials at FDA and other government agencies that "effectiveness wasn't everything. I may spend the '80s telling people that maybe safety isn't everything." She argued that there was a tendency in the women's health movement to consider safety to be the most important thing, when "perhaps our lives are much more diverse than that." Although Luker was skeptical about technological quick fixes, she also questioned the safety of some of the "natural" methods of self-abortion promoted by feminist health groups and clinics. "There seems to be a tendency—now particularly—to look back at the 'good old days' with a sort of warm glow," when in fact most folk remedies were ineffective and some were deadly. The long-term safety and effectiveness of the self-help technique of menstrual extraction had not been demonstrated either. Furthermore, concerns about the safety of contraceptives assumed that there was an open and risk-free alternative of abortion, but that needed to critically examined too. For some women, abortion was not a "trivial event" but rather had significant psychological and sociological implications. Luker believed it was "perfectly rational" for a woman to accept the risks of hormonal contraception because she would prefer not to have an abortion, yet Luker felt that this had "been invalidated as a legitimate choice at times." More importantly, it was possible that abortion as a political alternative would disappear in the future.[4]

Luker was not exaggerating. During the 1970s and 1980s, religious conservatives successfully organized to impose a number of restrictions to abortion access on the state and federal level, most of which were upheld by the U.S. Supreme Court. The pro-life movement became increasingly militant as well. In 1987, anti-abortion activist Randall Terry performed his first "rescue" of an unborn child by convincing a woman about to enter an abortion clinic not to terminate her pregnancy. The following year, Terry created the group Operation Rescue that advocated nonviolent direct action, including protests and blockades of abortion clinics, in their struggle to protect the lives of the unborn. By the late 1980s, anti-abortion militancy turned vicious, resulting in bombings of a number of clinics around the country and the assassinations of abortion providers and clinic staff. These mounting threats to women's reproductive rights made finding a safe and effective method of back-up contraception more critical than ever.

A Way Out of the Abortion Quagmire

Social and political opposition to the legalization of abortion began almost immediately after the *Roe v. Wade* decision was handed down by the U.S. Supreme Court in 1973.[5] That same year, pro-life activists formed the National Right to Life Committee to overturn women's right to legal abortion. By the late 1970s, anti-abortion groups had convinced seventeen state legislatures and a number of members of Congress to support the Human Life Amendment to the U.S. Constitution, which would have protected the life of an embryo from the moment of conception. Although attempts to pass a constitutional amendment were unsuccessful, the pro-life movement convinced their supporters in Congress to pass the Hyde Amendment, which prohibited using Medicaid to fund abortions except in cases of rape, incest, or conditions that endangered the life of the mother.

During the 1980s, the Republican Party made the re-criminalization of abortion a centerpiece of its party platform at its national convention in 1980. This conservative movement was a key factor in the election of President Ronald Reagan and a conservative Republican majority to both houses of Congress in 1980. That same year, the U.S. Supreme Court ruled in *Harris v. McRae* that while government could not obstruct a woman's right to choose abortion, it did not have to remove social conditions, such as poverty, for which it was not responsible. The right-to-life movement was especially adept at eroding adolescent girls' access to legal abortion. In 1981, Senators Jeremiah Denton (R-AL) and Orrin Hatch (R-UT) sponsored the Adolescent Family Life Act (AFLA), which sought to promote abstinence-only programs to curb the high incidence of teenage pregnancy. Incorporated into Title XX of the Public Health Service Act, the AFLA prohibited federal funding of adolescent pregnancy-prevention programs that advocated, promoted, or encouraged abortion. Although abortion rights groups challenged the constitutionality of the AFLA, the U.S. Supreme Court upheld the law in the decision *Bowen v. Kendrick* (1988). The following year, the Court's decision in *Webster v. Reproductive Health Services* upheld a Missouri state law that imposed restrictions on abortion access including mandatory waiting periods and parental notification requirements for minors seeking abortion services. Most alarmingly, the Court came within one vote of overturning *Roe* completely.[6]

Abortion activists did their best to combat this steady erosion of abortion access in the United States. The organization behind pro-choice activism leading up to the *Roe* decision, the National Association to Repeal Abortion Laws, renamed itself the National Abortion Rights Action League (NARAL). Prior to the 1980 presidential and congressional elections, NARAL and its state affiliates organized a political strategy called Impact 80 to combat the Moral Majority's efforts to defeat pro-choice candidates. Unfortunately, Impact 80 proved no match to the religious right's political power, and the 1980 election saw not only the election of an anti-abortion president but the defeat of many prominent pro-choice senators such as George McGovern. This major setback forced NARAL to regroup and form Impact 80s, the goal of which was to continue their efforts to get pro-choice candidates elected to national office.[7]

At the same time, feminist health organizations formed by women of color and their supporters began to criticize NARAL's narrow focus on the single issue of abortion access at the expense of other issues that disproportionately affected non-white women living in poverty. Women of color were especially disturbed by the tendency of NARAL and other mainstream reproductive rights groups to play into economic arguments that promoted enhancing access to abortion and birth control as solutions to the problem of poverty. Although women of color challenged militant civil rights leaders' allegation that the birth control movement was an instrument of black genocide, they also argued that the approach of mainstream population groups contributed to involuntary sterilization and other coercive policies that disproportionately affected women of color. A week after the Supreme Court issued its decision in *McRae,* upholding the constitutionality of the Hyde Amendment, representatives from various women's rights and feminist health groups formed the Committee for Abortion Rights and Against Sterilization Abuse (CARASA) to challenge conservative attacks on abortion and demand a more inclusive approach to women's reproductive rights. Members of CARASA insisted that reproductive rights be linked with other material conditions affecting women in poverty such as housing, income, and child care. For these women, reproductive freedom meant not only the right to limit their fertility, but also the right to reproduce regardless of race or income level.[8]

NARAL's political action director, Marie Bass, was on the front lines of the complex abortion politics of this period. Bass found her work for NARAL increasingly dissatisfying because of the way in which the abortion issue "had been appropriated by shallow, insensitive, and opportunistic politicians." Bass found that congressional candidates—"usually male, but not always"—formed their position on abortion according to "how the political winds in their state or district were blowing." Bass was especially discouraged by the fate of former congresswoman Geraldine Ferraro during her historic run for vice president in 1984. Ferraro was condemned by Cardinal John O'Connor "for her audacity, as a Catholic woman, to espouse a position on abortion that contradicted the Church." Meanwhile, pro-choice Catholic men (e.g., Mario Cuomo and Ted Kennedy) were given a pass. "Evidently, men could be indulged in a little waywardness, but a Catholic woman—never!" Throughout the 1980s, sporadic bombings and other incidence of violence aimed at abortion clinics led to a steady decline in the number of doctors willing to perform abortions. The situation was especially dire for poor women, since Medicaid would not cover abortions in most cases. To Bass, "the 'right' to an abortion was becoming a hollow legal shell having nothing to do with the ability to obtain one."[9]

Around the same time, Bass heard of a new abortifacent drug called RU 486 (mifepristone), which was in the process of being approved for market in France. She also learned of a small trial of RU 486 in United States by Dr. David Grimes of the University of Southern California, sponsored by the Population Council. Grimes found that eighty-five out of one hundred women given the drug to terminate an early pregnancy had a complete abortion.[10] The drug had to be taken within the first five to seven weeks of pregnancy in order to be effective. There was also some evidence that since RU 486 was an anti-progestin compound, it could also be used as a form of postcoital contraception. Bass thought that perhaps this new drug "was a way out of the quagmire of the abortion issue" since it would take abortion "out of the political arena and put the decision back in the hands of women and medical practitioners, where it belonged."[11]

Bass recruited other reproductive rights activists to support her efforts to bring RU 486 to the United States. Sarah Weddington, one of the lead attorneys in the *Roe v. Wade* case, endorsed Bass's work. Weddington helped raise awareness about RU 486 as she toured the country speaking with other abortion rights activists.[12] In 1987, Bass formed a political consulting firm with Joanne Howes, a former senior analyst in Planned Parenthood's national office. Bass, Howes, and former NARAL executive director Nanette Falkenberg obtained a grant from the Sunnen Foundation in St. Louis to conduct a survey of attitudes toward RU 486 among doctors and scientists involved in new drug research; leaders of family planning, pro-choice, and population organizations; officials at the National Institutes of Health and the FDA; members of women's health organizations and consumer groups; drug company representatives; and members of Congress and their political aides. The survey found there was tremendous support for this drug. Healthcare professionals believed that RU 486 and other progesterone antagonists could radically alter the field of reproductive medicine and dramatically change the politics of the abortion issue. At the same time, there was extreme pessimism about whether the drug could actually be approved and marketed in the United States. Not only was the political climate dismal for pursuing drugs pertaining to abortion or contraception, the chilling effect of lawsuits and congressional hearings involving various contraceptive drugs and devices made the pharmaceutical industry unwilling to invest in developing new products in this area.[13]

The survey report concluded that Bass, Howes, and Falkenberg should use these findings as the basis for a public information and education campaign that would encourage research on RU 486 and convince one or more drug companies to test and potentially market the drug in the United States.[14] They believed that without a concerted effort to promote the drug, the status quo regarding new contraceptives would go unchallenged. Risk-adverse drug companies would be reluctant to invest in developing a drug product, and anti-abortion organizations would be able to bar RU 486 from the United States.[15]

This public education campaign became even more urgent during the summer and fall of 1988, as anti-abortion groups' campaign against RU 486 intensified. The National Right to Life Committee sent letters to the French ambassador in Washington and to the American consulate in Paris, persuading them to raise concerns about the drug with French government officials. It was also clear that anti-abortion leaders in the United States were organizing demonstrations against the drug in Paris and disruptions of stockholders meetings for Roussel Uclaf, the French manufacturer of the drug. On October 26, 1988, the drug company announced that it was suspending distribution of RU 486 in response to right-to-life activities and threats of a worldwide boycott of the company. Roussel's decision led to an international public outcry. At a meeting of the World Congress of Gynecology and Obstetrics in Rio de Janeiro, healthcare professionals from around the world denounced the drug company's decision, declaring that RU 486 was "the most significant health advance for women since the birth control pill." Various pro-choice and family planning groups, such as Planned Parenthood, NARAL, the Alan Guttmacher Institute, the National Abortion Federation, the World Health Organization, and Catholics for Free Choice, all expressed outrage at Roussel's decision. On October 28, the French health minister ordered Roussel to resume manufacture and distribution of the drug in France, stating that once the government had approved the drug, "RU 486 became the moral property of women, not just the property of the drug company."[16]

Meanwhile, efforts by reproductive rights activists on behalf of pro-choice candidates during the elections of 1988 were unsuccessful. That year saw the victory of President George H. W. Bush and Vice President Dan Quayle, both strong opponents of abortion. It also saw the defeat of important congressional abortion rights supporters such as Senator Lowell Weicker of Connecticut.[17] This made the climate for pro-choice activism even chillier.

Bass, Howes, and Falkenberg realized they needed to do something to counteract this trend toward restricting women's reproductive rights. They met with Sharon Camp from the Population Crisis Committee, who was interested in promoting RU 486 as a way of dealing with the shocking rate of maternal mortality and septic abortions in the developing world.[18] Although Camp came from a mainstream population organization, her views on women and population issues departed radically from many other experts in the field. Camp believed that support for population issues during the Johnson and Nixon administrations was for the wrong reasons, especially the notion that overpopulation contributed to international terrorism and domestic political unrest. Camp, in contrast, came to the population movement through concerns about the impact of human population growth on the environment as well as an interest in promoting women's rights around the world. Camp recalled, "I was interested in saving the planet and in promoting equal opportunity for women and thought that both of those ends could be best achieved by giving women real reproductive choice."[19]

In late November 1988, Bass, Howes, and Camp organized a meeting to discuss how to bring RU 486 to the United States. They invited representatives from various organizations committed to reproductive rights, including NARAL, Planned Parenthood, the International Women's Health Coalition, the National Women's Health Network, the Boston Women's Health Book Collective, the National Black Women's Health Project, the Population Crisis Committee, and the Food and Drug Administration Center for Drug Evaluation and Research. Bass recalled, "While we were far from certain at the time as to what exactly we were doing, we agreed to form something with the rather mysterious name of the Reproductive Health Technologies Project." Although everyone at the meeting was pro-choice, they had widely differing opinions about RU 486.[20]

Loretta Ross, director of Women of Color Programs for the National Organization for Women, drew on her own experience to stress both her commitment to reproductive choice and her concerns about rushing new technologies to market. Ross was one of thousands of women who had suffered serious complications from using the Dalkon Shield: at age twenty-three, she decided to use the IUD while a student at Howard University because, she said, "I was not what they call a good contraceptor, because I'd just forget the things." After becoming pregnant and miscarrying, Ross decided she was a good candidate for the Dalkon Shield. At first, Ross did not suffer any of the usual menstrual difficulties associated with Dalkon Shield use. She recalled, "I thought I'd been blessed. I thought it was the greatest birth control, effortless, thoughtless, birth control." Unfortunately, the Dalkon Shield had a design flaw that made it easy for bacteria to enter the uterus. Three years after the device was implanted, Ross acquired a severe case of peritonitis and doctors performed a total hysterectomy to save her life.[21]

Ross observed that many supporters of RU 486, "in their panic and desperation for more birth control options, have compromised their once-vigilant concern for women's health." Ross warned that this "atmosphere of excitement about a new option" had led some to trivialize or dismiss outright possible drug risks. "Women should have learned from our experiences with noninvasive treatments such as DES and the birth control pill," Ross noted, "but in this struggle we have sometimes overlooked our history of being victimized by medical 'solutions.'"[22]

Judy Norsigian of the Boston Women's Health Book Collective pointed to earlier examples of racism and coercion in population control policy. She asked whether bringing RU 486 to the United States would replicate this prior history. She also raised the issue of whether women in rural areas would have access to emergency healthcare in case of drug complications such as prolonged bleeding.[23]

Despite these differences, most of the participants left the meeting with the consensus that they needed to do something to combat anti-choice groups' aggressive campaign against RU 486 and reproductive rights more generally.[24] In 1989, the Reproductive Health Technologies Project (RHTP) developed a media campaign and information kit on RU 486 to disseminate information about the drug and created a network of various women's organizations and other groups to receive feedback on women's reactions about RU 486 and other reproductive technologies.[25] Bass and Howes hoped that this media campaign would not only serve to combat the erroneous information spread by the anti-abortion movement but also provide a foundation for other new reproductive technologies.[26]

Yet as a group made up almost entirely of white women, the organization realized that, however well meaning, they could not represent the interests of all women. In order to include a diverse range of perspectives, the RHTP invited prominent women of color to join the board of directors. This included Julia Scott of the National Black Women's Health Project (NBWHP); Luz Alvarez Martinez of the National Latina Health Organization, physician-historian Vanessa Northington Gamble; and Helen Rodriguez-Trias, a physician of Puerto Rican heritage who was president of the American Public Health Association.[27] Rodriguez-Trias had been a strong advocate for reproductive rights for women of color since the 1970s and was a founding member of CARASA. Gamble worked on the history of race and gender issues in American medicine and public health. She believed that it was important for the RHTP "to acknowledge is that the needs and wishes of women are diverse and that we must take issues of differences in race, ethnicity, and class into account." Scott was a registered nurse whose activism centered around preventive medicine and empowering women of color. Scott "felt strongly that unless and until women of color can control their fertility, we cannot take advantage of other opportunities (i.e., affirmative action programs, employment, education and training, etc.) that could ultimately improve the quality of life for ourselves, our families and our communities." A key issue for Scott was "access to complete information and quality services," which would allow "a woman to make informed decisions and choices that are best for her and not for the convenience and approval of healthcare provider or policy makers." Another major concern for Scott was "the ever widening communications gap between women of color and the broader women's, scientific and health community. Historically new methods of contraception are targeted to low income women of color first, yet their voices are not sought or heard regarding the impact of these new drugs and devices in their lives." Scott hoped that her presence on the board would provide NBWHP with "an opportunity to learn more about these new technologies and the ability to engage in dialogue with others to explore the ways the new technology can improve and broaden the contraceptive choices for all women, especially low income women of color." More importantly, her input provided "an opportunity to share with the broader health, research and scientific community, information regarding the concerns and experiences of low income and poor women of color and the unique way reproductive technology impacts their lives." Scott felt that "by sharing and discussing information on the positive technical application of new technology as well as its potential for punitive and coercive use on low income women of color," the RHTP could "identify ways we can resolve our differences and support a common agenda that includes and empowers all women."[28]

The newly constituted board elected Sharon Camp of Population Action International as its chair. At their first meeting in July 1992, board members discussed what other reproductive technologies they wanted to support. They soon found that postcoital contraception was another issue on which they could find common ground.[29]

Breaking the Conspiracy of Silence

On January 5, 1994, ABC World News broadcast an edition of the *American Agenda* on the "morning-after pill," which the program dubbed "one of the best-kept secrets of the United States." Gary Stewart, director of Planned Parenthood in Northern California, claimed that "it's almost like there's been a conspiracy of silence" on the issue of emergency contraception. The problem started with pill manufacturers, who did not market oral contraceptives as "morning-after pills" because the FDA had not approved them for that purpose. The FDA's deputy commissioner Mary Pendergast told ABC News that the agency had approached drug companies suggesting that they submit applications to the FDA to approve the Yuzpe method as an indication for oral contraceptives, but none were interested. Manufacturers told the FDA that they were not willing to spend the time and money on an application process that would take years and result in the sale of only a few pills for emergencies. In addition, anti-abortion activists had used a provision of the Hyde Amendments to stop federally funded clinics from informing women that birth control pills could be used as postcoital contraceptives. The one place where the technology was relatively well known was on many college campuses. Health centers such as the one at the University of California, Davis, made their own postcoital contraceptive kits and used peer counselors to instruct young women on when and how to use them. One student interviewed for the story was grateful the pills existed but admitted they were not a substitute for good judgment: "You have to take responsibility in advance. . . . [B]irth control is not something to be thought about after." The report concluded that despite the controversy about postcoital contraceptives, there was an "emerging consensus" that "women should no longer be kept in the dark about this option."[30]

The ABC story was part of the RHTP's nationwide public education campaign to spread the word about the Yuzpe method. The idea for this initiative came from RHTP board member Felicia Hance Stewart, who described her "do-it-yourself" (DIY) approach to providing the Yuzpe method to her clients. Stewart said that she cut up packets of oral contraceptives and placed the Yuzpe regimen dosage in an envelope along with typed instructions on how and when to use the pills for postcoital contraception. Stewart gave these DIY envelopes to all her patients who came for birth control and reproductive health screening, telling them that this was a back-up method of contraception. Marie Bass thought this DIY strategy was fantastic and decided that this would be the next reproductive technology that the organization would promote.[31]

In 1993, the RHTP organized the Postcoital Contraceptives Task Force in order to publicize the Yuzpe method in the United States. The group believed it was especially important that women know about this option given the shortage of abortion providers and growing restrictions on abortion rights. The group also decided that as part of their awareness campaign they had to settle on a precise terminology for the technology. Although "morning-after pill" was catchy, they believed it also had "negative associations" and was not accurate since more than one pill was used and the method worked up to seventy-two hours after unprotected intercourse. Postcoital contraception was not easily understood or said by the average consumer. "Emergency contraceptive pills" was chosen as the best option since the word "emergency" communicated that this was "not a contraceptive for regular use." The Task Force and the RHTP Executive Board raised concerns about the potential for overuse of emergency contraception, a problem that could have added significance for teenagers with contraindications for oral contraceptives. They also remained divided about whether to make oral contraceptives, emergency or otherwise, available without a prescription. The board agreed, however, that safety concerns about emergency contraception needed to be put in the larger context of the abortion debate, which was making safe and affordable abortion increasingly unavailable to many American women.[32]

Members of the Task Force on Emergency Contraception believed that once women knew about and asked for this birth control method, pharmaceutical companies and healthcare providers were likely to respond to these requests. According to Gamble, emergency contraception was "a fundamental right to know issue. We have a way of reducing the need for abortion, and we are keeping that information hidden. It's time to let women in on the secret so that they can make their own informed decisions."[33] In 1994, the Task Force received the endorsement of Surgeon General Joycelyn Elders, who met with FDA commissioner David Kessler to discuss how to increase dissemination of information about emergency contraception.[34] The Task Force developed an information packet and distributed this to reproductive health organizations, public officials, and the press. They wrote sample resolutions on emergency contraception for various professional organizations, such as the Association of Reproductive Health Professionals and the American College of Obstetrics and Gynecology. The organization sent press kits to major news outlets, healthcare professionals, and professional associations to try to spread information about emergency contraception.[35] The RHTP helped place dozens of articles about how to assemble emergency contraception from birth control packages in popular women's magazines and national newspapers and ensured that the technology received prominent coverage on network news programs and the youth-oriented cable channel MTV.[36]

Word about the DIY method was further spread by activist-clinicians in college health centers and independent abortion clinics who created kits, postcards, and patient information sheets on the technology.[37] Renee Chelian of Northland Family Planning in Detroit recalls that when the clinic first began offering emergency contraceptive pills to all patients, she created "oops cards"—bright yellow postcards with the Os printed very large and condoms taped inside them. In addition, the cards contained information about a "second chance at preventing pregnancy" if a condom broke or one had unprotected intercourse. The cards listed the clinic's phone numbers and locations and were given to all patients who came in for abortions, pregnancy tests, ultrasounds, and other reproductive health services. The clinic also distributed the cards in bars in the Detroit area and had an independent record shop give out the cards on Valentine's Day. One year the clinic also made HOHOHO cards for Christmas and included not only information on emergency contraception, but also ways to show love without having sexual intercourse.[38] Planned Parenthood's legal council and insurer had accepted Stewart's protocol in 1988, officially clearing the way for affiliates to administer this treatment it to clients without fear of legal repercussions.[39] The DIY method of emergency contraception was also popularized in self-published feminist 'zines during the early 1990s.[40]

In 1995, James Trussell, Felicia Hance Stewart, and Robert Hatcher published *Emergency Contraception: The Nation's Best-Kept Secret,* which included information on which brands of birth control pills could be used for emergency contraception; the proper dosage for each brand; and a directory of providers and healthcare facilities where women could find emergency contraception.[41] The book was not widely distributed, however, and the provider directory soon became out of date. Trussell and the RHTP took the publicity campaign to the World Wide Web by launching an English- and Spanish-language emergency contraception website (http://opr.princeton.edu/ec/). Realizing that access to the Internet was still limited for many people, they also created an emergency contraception hotline (1–888-NOT-2-LATE) to provide information on how and where to get emergency contraception. To advertise the hotline, RHTP created a multimedia public education campaign in several major cities, including Chicago, Los Angeles, San Diego, and Seattle. This campaign included postcards, posters, advertisements on billboards and buses, and public service announcements on radio and television.[42]

Some reproductive health experts had so much faith in the DIY method that they proposed making oral contraceptives available over-the-counter so that women could more easily assemble the emergency contraceptive regimen on their own. In the fall of 1992, Trussell, Stewart, Hatcher, and Felicia Guest published an editorial in *Family Planning Perspectives* entitled "Emergency Contraceptive Pills: A Simple Proposal to Reduce Unwanted Pregnancies." The article argued that making oral contraceptives available without a prescription would be more effective than providing emergency contraceptive kits at family planning clinics. The authors believed that an even better method would

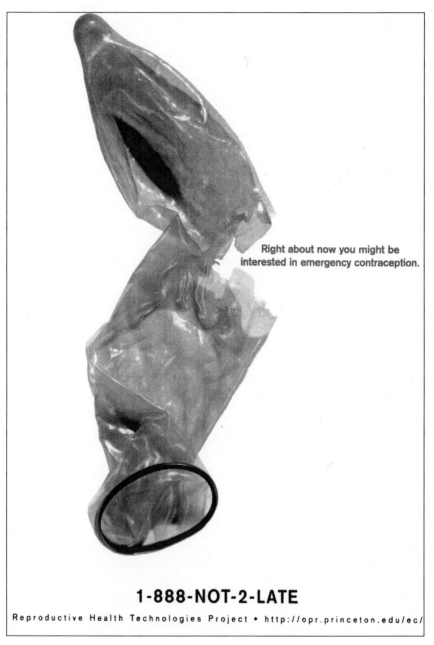

Right about now you might be
interested in emergency contraception.

1-888-NOT-2-LATE

Reproductive Health Technologies Project • http://opr.princeton.edu/ec/

Postcard from public awareness campaign by Reproductive Health Technologies Project,
1997. Courtesy of National Library of Medicine.

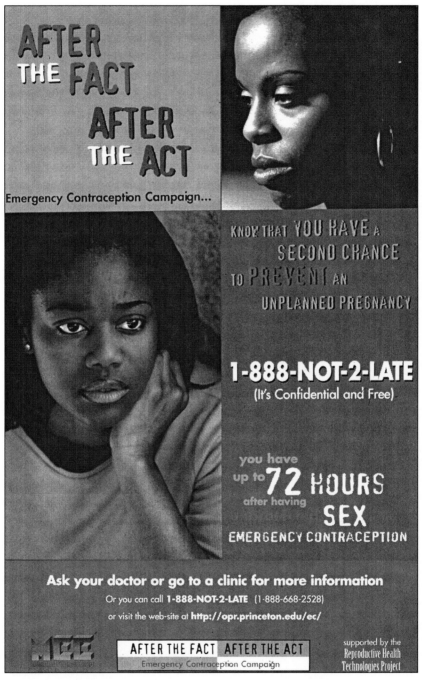

Poster from public awareness campaign by Reproductive Health Technologies Project, 1997. Courtesy of National Library of Medicine.

be to sell contraceptive pills packaged for emergency contraception use in vending machines. This could not be done without changing U.S. law, since birth control pills could not be sold without a prescription. However, the authors claimed that the benefits of current drug policy—protection of women with contraindications for hormonal contraceptives—were outweighed by the financial costs of visiting a physician as well as the human cost of unwanted pregnancy.[43]

The conservative daily newspaper the *Washington Times* quickly picked up this story, reporting, "While pro-lifers battle to keep the French abortion pill, RU 486, out of this country, it has largely gone unnoticed that other morning-after medications are being sold here legally." Not surprisingly, anti-abortion groups strenuously opposed the "simple proposal" of the making oral contraceptives available over-the-counter. Bob Marshall, a researcher for the American Life League, accused the authors of "abusing their medical knowledge" by advocating the use of oral contraceptives for emergency contraception when the FDA had not approved the drugs for such use.[44]

However, it was not just pro-life groups who were concerned about making oral contraceptives available without a prescription. Boston Women's Health Book Collective cofounder Judy Norsigian also pleaded, "Don't make the pill easier to acquire." Screening for contraindications for pill use should be more strenuous, not less, she argued. Data on the long-term effects of pill use was still inconclusive, she noted, especially for women who started taking the pill during adolescence.[45] Furthermore, feminist health groups and consumer activists were disturbed that a major pharmaceutical company was a key player in the drive to make oral contraceptives available without a prescription. The *Wall Street Journal* reported that an FDA open hearing on over-the-counter (OTC) status for oral contraceptives scheduled for February 1993 was backed by R. W. Johnson Pharmaceutical Research Institute, the research division of the research arm of Ortho Pharmaceutical Corporation, which manufactured the top-selling oral contraceptive brand, Ortho-Novum. Feminist health activists and representatives from consumer protection organizations charged that the pharmaceutical giant had pressured the FDA to organize the meeting so hastily that opponents of nonprescription status for oral contraceptives had insufficient time to prepare their arguments. Sidney Wolfe, director of the Public Citizen's Health Research Group, charged that the pill was "too potent a drug for over-the-counter." Wolfe argued that removing the prescription requirement would increase the use of the pills by women at risk for serious side effects. Cindy Pearson, program director for the National Women's Health Network, observed, "A birth control prescription is the poor woman's ticket to health care." Women who visited a birth control clinic not only received a prescription for contraceptives, but were also screened for sexually transmitted diseases, high blood pressure, cancer, and other health problems. Furthermore, Medicaid would not cover nonprescription birth control pills, forcing women to pay out of pocket for contraceptives they had previously received at little to no cost. Physicians and other health providers would lose the opportunity to counsel patients about the proper use and side effects of oral contraceptives. Adolescents were especially apt to discontinue use if they encountered uncomfortable side effects. Finally, healthcare professionals were concerned that making the pill available over the counter would make it less likely that women would be screened for STIs, leading to further spread of these diseases.[46] The BWHBC, along with the National Women's Health Network and the National Black Women's Health, concluded that "at this time it is not [a] good idea to make oral contraceptives available without prescription."[47] As a result of these protests, the FDA cancelled the proposed hearing on over-the-counter oral contraceptives.[48]

Nevertheless, the RHTP Task Force was successful in convincing the National Women's Health Network to reverse its long-standing opposition to emergency contraceptive pills. The Network's new position grew out of dialogue among women's health groups about RU 486 and the possibility of making oral contraceptives available without a prescription. Cindy Pearson served on the RHTP board of directors and represented the network's ongoing commitment "to the principles of lay women's involvement in health decisions, both in the exam room and in policy-making." She observed that the network had opposed approval of the hormonal contraceptives Depo Provera and Norplant because of unresolved safety issues and concerns about the disproportionate use of these drugs at clinics serving low-income women.[49] The network also believed that while the health risks of oral contraceptives had declined dramatically since they were first introduced, the remaining dangers were high enough that the group remained strongly opposed to over-the-counter approval for these drugs. At the same time, sufficient evidence about the safety and effectiveness of Yuzpe method had accumulated that the network was willing to "cautiously support its use." More importantly, increasing restrictions on abortion and access to federally funded birth control under Presidents Ronald Reagan and George H. W. Bush convinced the network that it needed to help ensure that women had access to emergency contraception when other birth control methods failed.[50]

This decision by the NWHN represented a major rapprochement between the organization and mainstream population control groups, representatives from the pharmaceutical industry, and members of more moderate women's health advocacy groups. Historically, the NWHN had been critical of the FDA's approval of high-dose estrogen regimes for contraception and hormone replacement therapy. NWHN was the first to protest the use of DES as an emergency contraceptive during the 1970s, and it continued to pressure the FDA to remain diligent in its oversight of postcoital use of other estrogen compounds. This shift in the NWHN's policy toward emergency contraception was a reaction to the escalating militancy and violence of the anti-abortion movement. In addition, many of the reproductive health professionals and population experts who advocated emergency contraception had adopted the women's rights framework advanced by the NWHN and other feminist health organizations. This led to the creation of what Sharon Camp called a "progressive community" that combined groups that historically had been at odds with each other.[51]

Thus, like the anti-rape movement before it, emergency contraception became a bridge issue between liberal feminists, radical feminists, and women of color. At the same time, changes were happening in Washington to create a more favorable climate for advancing a women's reproductive rights agenda. These shifts would lay the groundwork for a concerted effort by reproductive health professionals and feminist consumer activists to bring FDA-approved emergency contraceptives to the American market.

Chapter 6

Mainstreaming Emergency Contraception

On April 10, 1997, the popular medical drama television show *ER* included a brief scenario in which emergency room nurse Carol Hathaway (Julianna Margulies) treats a teenaged college student in the emergency room's free clinic. The young woman had been drugged with the sedative Rohypnol (aka "ruffies") and date raped at a party the night before. Hathaway gives the frightened young woman an emergency contraception kit and instructs her how to use it.[1] Although emergency contraception had been covered extensively by the press and network news programs during the 1990s, this was the first time it was featured prominently in a prime-time, major network television program.

It was fitting that this scenario appeared in a television series about the lives and loves of professionals in emergency medicine since the first uses of emergency contraception were for the treatment of rape victims in the emergency room at Yale–New Haven Hospital. By the 1990s, emergency contraception had become part of the standard of care for rape victims. In addition, the general public was becoming increasingly familiar with the fact that rape included not only assault by strangers but also date rape by boyfriends and male acquaintances. Yet emergency contraception was not well known even among those in the healthcare professions. In a survey conducted in 1995, the Kaiser Family Foundation (KFF) found that among the three hundred obstetrician-gynecologists surveyed, 77.5 percent reported that they were very familiar with postcoital contraceptive pills and 22.0 percent said they were somewhat familiar with them. The survey found that physicians seldom made women aware of this back-up method of birth control and, in those few cases, did so in response to an emergency rather than as part of regular contraceptive counseling. As a result, only 47 percent of the women surveyed indicated that they had heard of emergency contraception, and few of those had actually used it to prevent unwanted pregnancy.[2] Even students at colleges and universities where the DIY (do–it-yourself) method was readily available remained unaware that this technology existed. In an interview with the *New York Daily News,* Jasmine Brown, a student at Johnson C. Smith University in North Carolina, said that as an educated woman she knew all about birth control methods such as the Pill, Depo-Provera, and condoms, but told a reporter incredulously, "What's ECP [emergency contraceptive pill]? . . . How come we don't know about it?"[3]

The *ER* storyline was part of a larger effort by the various organizations in the 1990s to bring knowledge about emergency contraception into the mainstream. Early in 1997, the KFF approached NBC executives and the producers of *ER* with the idea of featuring emergency contraception in an episode of the hit series. The foundation chose *ER* as a vehicle for publicizing emergency contraception because of its enormous popularity (an average of thirty-four million viewers watched the show each week) and because the topic fit naturally within the series' subject matter. Prior to the episode's airing, independent researchers interviewed four hundred of the show's regular viewers about their knowledge of how to prevent unwanted pregnancy after unprotected intercourse. A week following the broadcast, over three hundred more viewers were interviewed. According to the survey, the percentage of *ER* viewers who knew about emergency contraception immediately following the broadcast was 17 percent greater than before viewing the show. This heightened awareness proved temporary, however: when interviewed two and a half months later, the number of viewers who reported they knew about emergency contraception had fallen back to 50 percent. The foundation concluded that the 17 percent of viewers who gained new information about contraception from the episode may not have retained it.[4]

Women who searched for emergency contraception at their local pharmacy were disappointed since there was no official product available to consumers. Instead, healthcare providers were still relying on the old DIY method of creating emergency contraceptive kits by cutting up and repackaging oral contraceptive pills with instructions on how to use them after unprotected intercourse. An advantage of the DIY approach was that health services and providers could remain under the radar of anti-abortion groups. In addition, women who learned about the DIY method through women's magazines, television coverage, or the Internet could assemble the regimen on their own using existing packages of oral contraceptives.[5]

Between 1995 and 1998, the Pacific Institute for Women's Health and Kaiser Permanente of Southern California attempted to professionalize the DIY method by conducting a million-dollar demonstration project financed by the David and Lucile Packard Foundation, the John Merck Fund, the Wallace Global Fund, and an anonymous donor. For this project, Kaiser Permanente's California Regional Pharmacy Operations Group repackaged oral contraceptives for use as emergency contraceptives and made these kits available to clients at Kaiser facilities throughout the San Diego area. It also created a media campaign to raise awareness about emergency contraception. The Program for Appropriate Technology in Health (PATH) created training materials for practitioners and educational materials for patients. The American College of Obstetricians and Gynecologists (ACOG) also gave professional legitimacy to the DIY method by creating practice guidelines for its members. PATH and KFF combined materials from the San Diego demonstration project and the ACOG practice guidelines to produce an information packet entitled *Emergency Contraception: Resources for Providers.* This source was endorsed by twelve major medical organizations, including the American Medical Association, and distributed to over fifty thousand healthcare providers around the country.[6]

Despite these promotional efforts, awareness of emergency contraception remained low. A 1997 survey indicated that only 11 percent of women of reproductive age had heard of emergency contraception. Even providers who knew about emergency contraception were not consistent about getting the word out to their patients: only 10 percent of those surveyed in 1997 indicated that they routinely counseled patients about this contraceptive option.[7]

Advocates for emergency contraception believed that the best way to spread knowledge about this method was to persuade pharmaceutical companies in the United States to manufacture and market a dedicated product designed specifically and exclusively for emergency contraception. According to James Trussell, the lack of a dedicated product packaged and labeled specifically for emergency contraception was the most significant barrier to more widespread use of this contraceptive method.[8] Other advocates for emergency contraception believed they had to do more than simply repackage regular birth control pills. Sharon Camp argued that cutting up packages of birth control pills and putting them in envelopes with mimeographed instructions "didn't look like real medicine." In order to legitimize this contraceptive method, she said, there needed to be a specific product approved by FDA and packaged specifically for emergency contraception.[9] Persuading a drug company to create such a product would not be an easy task.

Fighting the Birth-Control Backlash

In a *New York Times* Sunday magazine article in 1990, contraceptive chemical engineer Roderick Mackenzie commented on the lack of contraceptive options for American women. Since the introduction of the contraceptive pill in 1960, the United States had fallen behind other countries in contraceptive research and development. The number of U.S. pharmaceutical companies involved in contraceptive research and development fell from nine in 1980 to only one, Ortho Pharmaceutical, in 1990. Some population experts blamed this "birth-control backlash" on an "unwitting coalition" of courtroom litigators, feminists, right-to-life groups, and religious activists. Mackenzie, who had once directed Ortho Pharmaceutical Corporation in Canada and the United States, said the situation was more complex. He heaped scorn on manufacturers who perpetuated the myth that feminist activism and a litigious climate were to blame for the lack of women's birth control options in the United States. The truth, he said, was that the cost of litigation was very small compared with potential sales of contraceptives. Rather, pharmaceutical companies were more interested in developing products for ulcers, cardiovascular disease, and other conditions that created high profits but did not carry with them "a sea of bad publicity endangering other drugs."[10]

Mackenzie was among the few professionals in the pharmaceutical industry willing to work with women's health groups to develop and market new contraceptive products. In 1984, he founded the company Gynopharma to manufacture and market the Copper-T intrauterine device in the United States at a time when other companies were unwilling to do so because of fears of lawsuits.[11] In 1989, Marie Bass asked Mackenzie to join the efforts of the newly formed RHTP "to focus on new drugs such as RU 486 and to jointly work to combat the anti-abortion campaign against them."[12] At congressional hearings held on December 5, 1991, Mackenzie testified on the use of RU 486 in other countries and the obstacles to approval and marketing in the United States. Mackenzie observed that there was "a crisis in contraception in the United States." Due to fears of litigation and protests from anti-abortion activists, most manufacturers had abandoned the contraceptive market in the United States. As a result, highly effective methods involving hormones or IUDs were not used as much in the United States as they were in Western Europe or other parts of the world.[13]

Congresswoman Patricia Schroeder (D-CO) blamed the dearth of contraceptive options for American women on the backlash against feminism and reproductive rights during the 1980s. Schroeder claimed that the National Institutes of Health had done virtually nothing in the area of contraceptive research since the 1960s because of fears about the abortion issue and pressure from the far right.[14] During the late 1980s and early 1990s, Schroeder and Congresswoman Olympia Snowe (R-ME) co-chaired the Congressional Caucus for Women's Issues. One of the main goals of the caucus was to put pressure on NIH to increase resources for women's health research. At the same time, Dr. Florence Haseltine, an obstetrician-gynecologist at NIH, organized fellow members of ACOG and other experts in women's health to demand more attention at NIH to gynecological research and women's health needs more generally. In 1990, Haseltine and her colleagues founded the Society for the Advancement of Women's Health Research (SAWR) to provide leadership on the issue of healthcare equity. That same year, SAWR and the Congressional Caucus requested that the General Accounting Office (GAO) conduct an audit of NIH procedures regarding women and clinical research. The GAO reported that NIH had made little progress in this area. The resulting outcry on Capitol Hill and in the national media led to important changes at NIH, including the creation of the Office of Research on Women's Health and the appointment of Dr. Bernadine Healy as director of NIH, the first woman to ever hold that post. Members of the Congressional Caucus introduced the Women's Health Equity Act, which not only included support for new research, but also improved access to healthcare and treatment for women.[15]

This growing support for women's health issues was evident at the FDA as well. Pressure from women's health advocates paved the way for the appointment of the agency's first female commissioner, Jane Henney, by President Bill Clinton.[16] Emboldened by these changes, various women's health groups came together to convince the FDA to reexamine its position on emergency contraception. On November 23, 1994, the Center for Reproductive Law and Policy (CRLP), with the support of the Packard Foundation, filed a citizen's petition on behalf of the American Medical Women's Association, the American Public Health Association, and Planned Parenthood of New York City, demanding that the FDA require the drug manufacturers Wyeth-Ayerst Laboratories and Berlex Laboratories to revise the patient package insert for oral contraceptives to include use as emergency contraception. Other women's health organizations, including the National Women's Health Network, the National Black Women's Health Project, the National Latina Health Organization, the National Women's Law Center, and Advocates for Youth, soon signed onto the petition. The CRLP petition claimed that the FDA had sanctioned "criminal misbranding" by manufacturers by failing to require all regimens that could safely and effectively prevent pregnancy on the package inserts. The petition demanded that the FDA require manufacturers to revise the indications for oral contraceptives so that American women and their healthcare providers could be fully informed about the emergency use of these contraceptives to prevent pregnancy.[17]

This petition represented a new development in the fraught relationship between the FDA and advocates for women's health. During the 1970s and 1980s, many leading feminist health activists claimed the agency was too careless in approving new drugs and devices for contraception. This lack of adequate oversight had led to a number of health disasters for women who used hormonal contraception. The citizen's petition filed by the CRLP was part of a larger movement by consumer activist groups—most notably, organizations dedicated to fighting AIDS—to increase the availability of new medical treatments by accelerating the drug approval process.[18] Like AIDS activists before them, the authors and supporters of the citizen's petition claimed that the FDA's inaction on the issue of emergency contraception was "an irresponsible abdication of its duty to safeguard the public health." Although numerous studies in Europe, Canada, and the United States had demonstrated that the Yuzpe method was as safe and effective as other indications for oral contraceptives, the FDA was deliberately endangering the health and lives of women by suppressing knowledge about this important contraceptive technology. The petition argued that because patient inserts for oral contraceptives failed to provide information on emergency contraception, these products were misbranded in violation of Section 502 of the Food, Drug, and Cosmetic Act of 1938. By condoning this mislabeling, the petition argued, the agency was in violation of its own regulations governing prescription drug labeling and the content of patient package inserts.[19]

The petition claimed that misbranding had serious consequences not only for women's health but for the practice of medicine in the United States. Although popular articles and coverage on national news programs had raised awareness about emergency contraception, most women did not know the recommended dosage and timing, contraindications, or side effects; nor did they know which brands of oral contraceptives were appropriate for emergency contraception. Thus, there was a significant danger that women would self-medicate without complete information and thereby endanger their health. This problem was especially dire in areas where women had limited access to physicians or could not obtain an appointment and prescription within the requisite seventy-two hours. If full information about emergency contraception were available on the package insert, these health risks would be greatly reduced. Furthermore, the failure of oral contraceptive manufacturers to label or publicize the postcoital use of their products, and the failure of the FDA to force manufacturers to do so, interfered with a woman's right to make an informed choice among legal, safe, and effective contraceptive methods. This interference, in turn, deprived women of their right to privacy in reproductive healthcare decision-making. Poor women and adolescents were disproportionately affected by these problems since they received reproductive care at Title X clinics that were forbidden to use oral contraceptives off-label for emergency contraception. Finally, mislabeling had a "chilling effect" on the practice of medicine. Although healthcare providers were free to prescribe approved drugs for unapproved uses, many were reluctant to do so because of fears of malpractice lawsuits. In addition, prevailing interpretation of U.S. drug law made it illegal for providers to inform non-patients, including other healthcare professionals, about "off-label" uses of drugs. This prevented practitioners from learning about emergency contraception and impinged on health professionals First Amendment rights to discuss and teach about a safe and effective off-label use of an approved drug.[20]

Because physicians were prohibited from disseminating accurate medical information about emergency contraception, volunteers and health educators at many university health clinics and rape crisis centers had developed informational pamphlets and flyers describing this birth control method. Although these documents were helpful in spreading knowledge about the technology, because they were produced without official physician participation, they subjected employees of university health clinics and rape crisis centers to charges of unauthorized practice of medicine.[21]

Testimony from healthcare practitioners emphasized the impact that FDA approval would have on use of emergency contraception. Barbara A. Nevergold and Colleen Brown from Planned Parenthood of Buffalo and Erie County told FDA commissioner David Kessler that "FDA recognition of the ECPs would represent a significant first step toward widespread awareness and use of ECP" as it would allow manufacturers and distributors to advertise this method of using birth control pills. It would also permit physicians to teach and train other healthcare providers about the proper emergency contraceptive regimen. Relabeling would also ensure that Title X clinics could use and be reimbursed for these pills, and it would legalize overseas use by the U.S. Agency for International Development and its grantees. Most importantly, they argued, "relabeling would put information about ECPs directly into the hands of each woman who has a prescription for oral contraceptives."[22] Gynecologist David Grimes, chief of the Department of Obstetrics, Gynecology, and Reproductive Sciences at San Francisco General Hospital, argued that the FDA was going against its own mandates to provide complete and accurate information on the patient package insert. He observed that it made "no sense from a public health standpoint" to include information about how oral contraceptives could give a woman lighter periods but not include the fact that pills could be used for emergency contraception. "The rest of the world looks to the U.S. as leader in medical research and technology," he argued. The omission of this information had a "chilling effect" not only on medical practice in the United States, but on postcoital contraceptive use around the world.[23]

Dr. Jane E. Hodgson of the Women's Health Center in Duluth, Minnesota, described her experience working at a Title X clinic from 1988 to 1992, where she found "the effect of FDA sanctioned mislabeling so inhibiting that I felt almost compelled to quit." Although the practice of off-label use of approved drugs was common, she felt that the current climate in the field of reproductive health did not offer "any leeway to deviate from the letter of FDA labeling, even when such labeling is wrong," especially in publicly financed clinics: "With family planning practitioners being shot, poisoned, fire-bombed and otherwise harassed, we cannot afford to open ourselves to even the possibility of frivolous lawsuits that will be costly and burdensome to defend by using drugs in any way not explicitly approved by the FDA." Hodgson found through her work at a school-based health clinic that teenagers were especially in need of emergency contraception because they were less likely to use contraceptives correctly, use them at time of first intercourse, or plan ahead. These facts about teen use indicated that practitioners needed a "free hand" in prescribing contraceptives to this age group. Hodgson also raised concerns about the FDA's inaction on emergency contraception for teenagers and older women who were raped. "Such women suffer additional trauma from the fear that they may conceive as a result of the rapes, and yet FDA inactivity hampers doctors from helping allay the fears of these women." Hodgson said that even her private practice was hindered by the FDA's failure to label birth control pills for emergency use. Hodgson encouraged her patients to educate themselves about the medications she gave them, but many of them worried when they saw that postcoital use was not an indication on the package inserts for oral contraceptives. "As a physician, I feel the integrity of my relationship with my patients is breached when FDA fails to enforce their own guidelines and causes my patients to doubt the advice I give them," Hodgson stated. "Even though they may need the medication to reduce their chances of pregnancy after unprotected intercourse, some of my patients have opted not to take the pills when they have learned that the indication has been omitted by the FDA." Although she said she could create her own labels for patients, Hodgson did not feel that "home-made labels, although more accurate than the currently available commercial ones blessed by the FDA, would be respected by other practitioners or even patients."[24]

In November 1995, the director of the FDA's Center for Drug Evaluation and Research (CDER), Janet Woodcock, informed the CRLP that while the agency agreed in principle that it had discretion to require that oral contraceptives be relabeled to include emergency use, the CDER declined to do so in this instance. However, the agency did decide it would be appropriate to discuss the issue with the Reproductive Health Drugs Advisory Committee at its next meeting.[25]

On June 28, 1996, the Reproductive Health Advisory Committee heard testimony from Dr. James Trussell, who discussed efficacy issues, and Dr. Elizabeth Barden, who discussed safety issues and the experience in her country, the United Kingdom, with emergency contraceptive pills. Dr. Stanley Zinberg read a statement on behalf of the American College of Obstetricians and Gynecologists, and Janet Benshoof, JD, summarized the arguments of the CRLP petition. Dr. Willa Brown spoke on behalf of the American Medical Women's Association. Following testimony from various organizations supporting emergency contraception, as well as prominent opponents such as the American Life League, the advisory committee voted unanimously that the Yuzpe method was 75 percent effective in preventing unwanted pregnancy and was safe enough to include in the patient package insert for oral contraceptives.[26] This was a highly unusual decision for the agency: never before had FDA made a decision about a drug in the absence of an application for a specific product from a particular manufacturer. Benshoof told the *Philadelphia Inquirer*, "They [FDA] stepped into a big void, because drug-makers would not change their labeling."[27]

In an interview with the *New York Times*, FDA deputy commissioner Mary Pendergast stated the agency was hoping that this decision would pave the way for greater access to emergency contraception by alleviating women's anxieties about using birth control pills for this purpose. Leslie Gruss, a Manhattan gynecologist, observed that while physicians had been using the Yuzpe method for years, the FDA's decision was "like the Good Housekeeping seal of approval" for practitioners.[28] It also meant that proponents of emergency contraception could be more aggressive in their efforts to raise awareness about this technology.

A Courageous Step

In March of 1997, the FDA published a notice in the *Federal Register* requesting that manufacturers submit supplemental new drug applications for emergency use for certain oral contraceptives.[29] "The best-kept contraceptive secret is no longer a secret," said FDA commissioner David A. Kessler in an interview for the *Washington Post* announcing this move. This was another unusual decision by the agency, as it was the first time that the FDA had invited companies to create and market a particular drug or device. Gloria Feldt, president of Planned Parenthood Federation of America, called the agency's decision "a bold step—a courageous step," because it would bring information about emergency contraception to far more women.[30]

The FDA's announcement was issued after futile efforts to convince a drug company to create a dedicated product for the Yuzpe method. Philip A. Corfman recalled that he and other FDA officials were "annoyed as hell" that major American contraceptive manufacturers they approached were not interested in producing an emergency contraceptive product. "All they had to do was take something they were already making, put it in another package, and market it," said Corfman.[31] Representatives from Wyeth Ayerst Laboratories, manufacturer of four of the oral contraceptive pills that could be used for the Yuzpe method, said the company had no interest in relabeling their pills for use as emergency contraceptives because they believed it was unprofitable and because liability concerns and threatened boycotts by abortion opponents made such a venture economically risky.[32]

Corfman finally asked Roderick Mackenzie to consider venturing into an area that other pharmaceutical manufacturers refused to touch. Mackenzie had just sold Gynopharma to Johnson & Johnson but wanted to continue his work making new contraceptive products available to American women. "I was wondering what I was going to do next," Mackenzie recalled. "So it was fortuitous that the FDA came to me and asked me to help make emergency contraceptives happen."[33] In 1995, Mackenzie created the company Gynetics specifically for the purpose of bringing a dedicated emergency contraceptive product to market. "In female reproductive medicine, you have to be very, very cautious," he told the *Philadelphia Inquirer.* "But you can do it, and you can protect your investors at same time."[34] Mackenzie funded the company entirely on his own until the FDA announcement in 1997 inviting new drug applications from manufacturers interested in creating an emergency contraceptive product. Mackenzie then began actively seeking investors for Gynetics. Mackenzie explained his motivations in an interview with *Fortune* magazine: "I started working in the oral contraceptive field at the very beginning of its existence," Mackenzie said. "It was very exciting, because despite getting adverse publicity, we felt a tremendous sense of doing good."[35]

When the FDA approached Mackenzie about developing an emergency contraceptive product, they told him "there was a very big public health need." Mackenzie found that the opportunity to prevent abortions and unintended pregnancies was compelling enough to accept the FDA's invitation. In November of 1997, he submitted a new drug application with the FDA for a product containing the same formulation and dosage as the Yuzpe method. On September 1, 1998, the FDA approved his application. Soon after, Gynetics, along with its manufacturing partner Barr Laboratories, released Preven Emergency Contraceptive Kit, the first FDA-approved emergency contraceptive product. The kit contained four combination birth control pills, a home pregnancy test, and a patient information guide. "Having the kit makes this whole process much simpler," noted Mackenzie. "It is simpler for the doctors to prescribe, it is simpler for the pharmacists to dispense, the instructions make it simple for a woman to use, the pregnancy test adds confidence, and just the right number of the right pills are there so there's no guessing."[36]

In October 1998, Gynetics launched a ten-million-dollar direct-to-consumer advertising campaign for Preven. This type of marketing was made possible by recent revisions of FDA policies regarding direct-to-consumer (DTC) activities for drug companies. By the late 1980s, the agency reversed its longstanding policy by allowing print advertising in newspapers and magazines aimed at the general public. In 1997, the FDA allowed advertising using broadcast media. The late 1990s also saw the growth of DTC advertising on the World Wide Web.[37] Print advertisements for Preven designed by Nelson Communications in New York City featured full-page, four-color advertisements in major magazines such as *Entertainment Weekly* and *People.* The advertisements showed an unmade bed with a tagline, "The condom broke. But my life stayed intact."[38] The campaign included radio spots in major metropolitan markets; coverage on national news programs on CBS, NBC, ABC, and PBS; and plugs by the popular advice show *Loveline* on MTV. The company also created its own toll-free hotline (1–888–PREVEN2) and website (www.preven.com).[39] When interviewed about the advertising campaign, Mackenzie said, "We wanted to design an ad that helps relieve a woman's sense of anxiety over the possibility of becoming pregnant due to contraceptive failure or sex without birth control. We also wanted to inform women that a new FDA-approved contraceptive option is now available that can help reduce their risk of an unintended pregnancy."[40]

Like other contraceptives, Preven was available at low cost to clients of federally funded family-planning clinics. Soon after the product was approved, Gynetics gave twenty-five thousand Preven kits to Planned Parenthood clinics to distribute to low-income women.[41] Gynetics also donated kits to Title X clinics and made them available at reduced cost to student health centers. However, women whose income was too high to use these facilities had to purchase the kit at the full cost of twenty dollars per kit. According to Mackenzie, Preven was more affordable than the DIY method, since it cost less than any oral contraceptive on the market. Previously, women had to buy an entire month's supply of oral contraceptives. The Preven kit simply contained the four pills required for emergency contraception, along with a pregnancy test and a patient information guide on how to use the product. Gloria Feldt, president of the Planned Parenthood Federation of America, admitted that Preven was "going to be expensive for some women, but for many women, it will be a product that they will be extremely pleased to pay that price for. It's important for women to have a choice of options."[42]

Doing It Ourselves

To Sharon Camp, having only one emergency contraceptive product on the market did not offer enough choice to American women. "Competition in the emergency contraception marketplace can only bode well for women," she observed after the release of Preven. There were over one hundred brands of oral contraceptives on the market, "so why should there only be one emergency contraceptive?" Camp asked. "The more companies that are out there advertising emergency contraception directly to the consumer and educating healthcare providers, the more likely it is that emergency contraception will become a standard part of reproductive health care." Competition would also bring down costs and possibly entice larger pharmaceutical companies to enter the market. Advertising of competing would further publicize emergency contraception. According to Alexander Sanger, president of Planned Parenthood of New York City, the result would be that "women are going to have choices, and will be able to make the choice that is best for them."[43]

Camp also believed that there were better methods of emergency contraception than Preven. Like other high-dose pills containing both estrogen and progestin, Preven caused severe nausea in about half the women who took it, causing one in five of these to vomit up the drug. Research conducted in China in the early 1990s indicated that pills consisting solely of the progestin compound levonorgestral were just as effective as the older Yuzpe method, with fewer side effects.[44] Camp had tried to convince Mackenzie that he should work on developing a levonorgestral product, but Mackenzie believed that he could get the Yuzpe method through the regulatory process at the FDA much sooner. Because the FDA had already endorsed the Yuzpe method, Gynetics was able to submit a new drug application without having to conduct new clinical trials. The same expedited process could not be done with the levonorgestral-only regimen since the FDA had never before considered this method of emergency contraception.[45]

In October of 1995, the Rockefeller Foundation convened a meeting of various groups interested in promoting emergency contraception as an alternative to unsafe abortion, especially in the developing world. Shortly after the meeting, those who attended the meeting formed the International Consortium for Emergency Contraception (ICEC). The consortium consisted of seven organizations: the Concept Foundation, International Planned Parenthood Federation, Pacific Institute for Women's Health, Pathfinder International, the Program for Appropriate Technology in Health, the Population Council, and the World Health Organization Special Programme of Research, Development, and Research Training in Human Reproduction (which was conducting a multisite international study of the use of the progestin compound levonorgestral as an emergency contraceptive).[46]

Coordinated by Sharon Camp, the ICEC set out to make emergency contraception an integral part of women's health around the world. The group worked with the Hungarian drug company Gideon Richter to get the company's levonorgestral product Postinor through the regulatory process and on the market in forty countries. The ICEC started with countries in the developing world, where access to safe abortion was minimal. According to Camp, while the ICEC was launching Postinor in developing countries, "it quickly became clear that if we weren't going to be promoting second-class medicine for third-world women, we needed to seek approval for the product in a major western-industrialized country." Since the FDA was "reputed to be the toughest [regulatory agency] in the world," Camp and other members of ICEC believed, "If we could get the product through the Food and Drug Administration that it would be validated as safe and effective all over the world, and it would accelerate the adoption of this new and improved product all over the world." Gideon Richter was not willing to bring the drug to the United States on its own but agreed to secretly supply the product to a U.S. pharmaceutical company.[47]

However, no drug company in the United States was willing to engage in marketing a product that was highly controversial and showed little promise of being profitable. Out of frustration, Camp decided to found her own pharmaceutical company, Women's Capital Corporation (WCC), in January 1997. Camp was inspired by conference called "Doing It Ourselves" organized by Eleanor Smeal of the Feminist Majority Foundation. The theme of the conference was this: "It's time for women to take charge. We've been waiting for men to do things for us too long and it, we all, in every aspect of life and business, it's time for women to take charge and do what women needed."[48]

This ethic of doing it ourselves had been central to the mission of feminist health groups since the 1960s. The WCC represented an extension of this philosophy to the development and marketing of new pharmaceutical products. According to Camp, the pharmaceutical industry "demonstrated the political instincts of celery," bending too easily to shifts in the political landscape and caving in too readily to pressure from conservative groups. Camp "wanted to try and find a way to get new products to market faster" and believed that her experience working with women's health and reproductive choice communities would help accelerate approval of new contraceptive technologies for women. Camp initially went to over 150 private equity firms to try to get funding for her company, but no one would provide financing, even ones that "were run by women who really wanted to get involved in this," because they felt it "was simply too risky and controversial for them." Instead, Camp turned to private nonprofit foundations dedicated to reproductive health for support. Investors included the Wallace Global Fund, the Compton Foundation, the Wallace Alexander Gerbode Foundation, the Packard Foundation, and the International Foundation for Family Health, as well as several Planned Parenthood affiliates.[49]

The creation of WCC represented what Lisa Wynn refers to as a "unique partnership" between feminist health activists, reproductive rights and reproductive health organizations, researchers, physicians, and private investors. Typically, pharmaceutical companies are viewed as "a corrupting, commercial influence on medical professionals and researchers." The history of WCC contradicts this stereotype in that it was a small pharmaceutical company founded and supported largely by activists and nonprofit organizations.[50] In order to create a focal point for advancing the cause of emergency contraception in the United States, these emergency contraceptive activists from ICEC and related organizations founded the American Society for Emergency Contraception (ASEC) in the fall of 1997 to specifically address U.S. policy and advocacy issues. The organization was especially intent on serving as a "watchdog for inaccurate or biased articles in the press" and "abuses of reproductive rights related to emergency contraception." The ASEC also aimed to circulate policy statements and guidelines to other organizations and to link members of the emergency contraception field through newsletters and an annual meeting.[51]

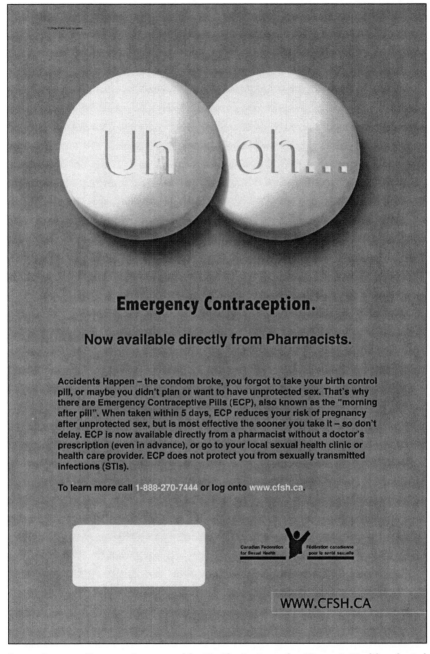

Image from media campaign created by Pacific Institute for Women's Health, adapted by Canadian Federation for Sexual Health. Courtesy of Canadian Federation for Sexual Health.

In 1998, the WCC applied to the FDA for approval of the levonorgestral product Plan B and submitted data on the safety and effectiveness of the drug, compiled by the World Health Organization (WHO) and other researchers affiliated with ICEC. The FDA approved the drug, but the agency's Labeling and Nomenclature Committee rejected the trade name because it thought it was "flippant" and had a "meaningless B suffix." Camp, however, insisted that the name had the "right public health message," that is, "when Plan A fails, you can go to Plan B." WCC appealed the decision and convinced CDER director Janet Woodcock to rule in their favor. Woodcock agreed with Camp that the phrase "Plan B" was a "useful public health method" because it implied "a sequence or order that emergency contraception should be a backup or emergency plan, not the primary method." Furthermore, the emergency contraception scenario was "unusual in that only the individual woman is in a position to recognize when Plan A fails and the need for emergency contraception is triggered. Therefore, it is of utmost importance that the individual consumer thoroughly understands the role and timing of intervention."[52]

Rather than follow Gynetics' strategy of direct-to-consumer marketing and distribution to major pharmacies, the WCC chose to initially market and distribute Plan B to facilities that prescribed and distributed contraceptives on-site—including college and university health services, Planned Parenthood, rape crisis enters, and Title X birth control clinics. According to Camp, WCC was "an outgrowth of a private/public consortium, so we have a very strong public-sector focus."[53] The WCC also had a very small marketing budget—slightly more than a quarter of a million dollars—and needed to spend it strategically. In 2002, the company enlisted DDB, an advertising company in Seattle, to launch its first major advertisement campaign, which was directed at sexually active college women. On Valentine's Day of that year, thirty college newspapers around the country featured ads and inserts with such slogans as "Accidents happen. That's why there's morning-after contraception" and "So many men. So many reasons to have backup contraception."[54]

Advocates for emergency contraception were not content to have dedicated products approved for prescription use only. They soon renewed their efforts to make emergency contraceptive pills available over the counter. Accomplishing this goal meant combating an increasingly chilly climate for women's reproductive rights in the new century.

Chapter 7

From Paternalism to Patient Empowerment

In a special issue on emergency contraception in 1999, the *Journal of the American Medical Women's Association* argued that the time had come to make emergency contraception available over the counter (OTC). The journal editors argued that the harm of keeping this method out of women's hands outweighed the potential risks of making emergency contraceptive pills more widely available by removing the prescription status. The article concluded that "the special paternalistic scrutiny accorded to contraceptive methods used by women be relaxed" and that emergency contraception join the ranks of other OTC drug products.[1]

Feminist health activists had been battling the medical profession's paternalistic treatment of women since the 1960s. The fact that this statement appeared in a medical journal written by and for women physicians demonstrated the extent to which activists had become insiders in the medical profession and brought with them the feminist health movement's perspective on reproductive rights. At the same time, the position on the balance between risk and safety had changed considerably. While health feminists in the 1970s argued that the morning-after pill was too dangerous to be on the market, by the early twenty-first century, women's health groups were arguing that emergency contraception was safe, effective, and less risky than unwanted pregnancy.

Advocates for emergency contraception were not the only ones who were seeking to make their drug available without a prescription. They were following the example of other drugs that had recently been switched to OTC status. This trend began in the 1970s and accelerated during the 1990s. There were thirty-nine prescription drugs switched to OTC between 1976 and 1989. In comparison, there were twenty such switches between 1990 and 1996. This dramatic increase in the availability of nonprescription drugs was partly the result of consumers who demanded a greater choice of OTC products. In addition, the Waxman-Hatch Act of 1984 gave manufacturers an economic incentive by giving manufacturers three years of marketing exclusivity if the OTC product contained the same formulation as the prescription version.[2] Applications for OTC status for a particular drug came from manufacturers, many of whom hoped to extend their patent protection and benefit from brand name recognition they had already established with a prescription-only product. Pharmacologist R. Wiliam Soller coined the term "OTCness" to describe this explosion in the availability of nonprescription drugs.[3] The growing self-care movement in 1990s prompted the FDA to take a closer look at the kinds of medications that should be considered appropriate for OTC use. These included not only emergency contraceptive pills, but also cholesterol-lowering drugs, diuretics, antihypertensive agents, asthma treatments, and regular oral contraceptives.[4] Proponents of emergency contraception joined this larger trend and began pressuring FDA to make this birth control method available without a prescription.

A Quiet Revolution

As noted in chapter 5, attempts to make emergency contraception available without prescription dated back to the early 1990s. Reproductive health experts at that time argued that selling oral contraceptives without a prescription would make it easier for women to use the Yuzpe method because they would not need to see a healthcare professional.[5] The supporters of OTC status for oral contraceptives claimed that keeping these drugs under physician control was no longer necessary and in fact treated women like children. They challenged the "common public perception" that women needed gatekeepers to help them select and teach them how to use birth control pills. They argued that this perception was a result of the prescription status itself, which encouraged patients "to be trusting and docile." Although they acknowledged that OTC status might lead to a decline in efficacy because women would not need to see a clinician and therefore would not receive counseling on how to use the product. Yet they also argued that prescription status created "significant obstacles to access," including costly initial visits and follow-ups to see a physician or nurse practitioner. In fact, prescription status itself discouraged use of oral contraceptives by implying that they were "unsafe." Removing the prescription requirement, they argued, would eliminate this barrier by signaling the drugs were indeed safe. Nonprescription status "would also stimulate direct advertising to women, creating another channel for consumers to learn about safe and effective" use of oral contraceptives.[6]

This argument in favor of patient empowerment was adopted by some officials at the FDA. Philip A. Corfman, director of the agency's Center for Drug Evaluation and Research, went so far as to argue, "'I think the pill is safer than aspirin and aspirin is available over the counter.'"[7] Corfman was so convinced that oral contraceptives were safe enough to be switched to nonprescription status that he scheduled a public hearing with the center's Fertility and Maternal Health Drugs Advisory Committee. Because of opposition from both anti-abortion groups and consumer activists, the FDA cancelled the public hearing and did not pursue the issue any further at that time.[8]

With the approval of two dedicated emergency contraceptive products, Preven and Plan B, the situation had changed. Advocates for OTC status for emergency contraception no longer had to promote the Yuzpe method and could now separate emergency contraception from the question of whether to make regular birth control pills available without a prescription.

The groundwork for an appeal to make emergency contraception available without a prescription was laid by a group of organizations in Washington State who used legislation permitting collaborative agreements between pharmacists and physicians as the basis for a demonstration project on emergency contraception in the Puget Sound area. These collaborative agreement laws allowed pharmacists to prescribe and dispense certain drug therapies. The two-year pharmacy access demonstration project, conducted between 1998 and 2000, was funded by the David and Lucile Packard Foundation and managed by the Program for Appropriate Technology in Health (PATH), working in partnership with the Washington State Board of Pharmacy, the Washington State Pharmacists Association, the University of Washington Department of Pharmacy, and Elgin/DDB, a public relations firm that had worked with the Reproductive Health Technologies Project to publicize the Yuzpe method of emergency contraception. The project gave training sessions for pharmacists to educate them about all aspects of emergency contraception and to help them set up collaborations with healthcare providers in their area. Elgin/DDB created print and radio advertisements informing women that pharmacists were prescribing emergency contraception and promoting the national telephone hotline and website for emergency contraception operated by the Reproductive Health Technologies Project.[9] Although anticipated protests from anti-abortion groups never materialized, most pharmacists chose not to have signs advertising emergency contraception in order to avoid controversy. This "quiet revolution" started by the Washington State demonstration project was successful enough that other states with pharmacist collaborative agreements began experimenting with pharmacy access programs for emergency contraception.[10]

Pharmacists were not always allies, however. When the FDA approved Preven, the retail giant Wal-Mart refused to stock the emergency contraceptive kits. Spokespersons from Wal-Mart claimed this was purely a business decision, but Planned Parenthood officials suspected that the company feared boycotts and protests from abortion opponents. Planned Parenthood threatened to launch a boycott of Wal-Mart, claiming that the company was deserting women living in areas where it had a monopoly on prescription drugs. Alexander C. Sanger, president of Planned Parenthood of New York City, said the organization thought it was unacceptable for Wal-Mart pharmacies not to carry Preven. Since Wal-Mart pharmacies were licensed by the states in which they operated, they were part of the public health system. Sanger argued it was "incumbent upon them to have available this time-sensitive medication." Marie Griffin, editor of the trade publication *Drug Store News,* argued that pharmacies "should not get involved in the sacred relationship between a physician and patient." Pharmacists for Life International disagreed with this position, claiming that a pharmacist had a right to refuse to fill a prescription that violated his or her moral beliefs. Despite reassurances from Gynetics that Preven was a contraceptive, not an abortion drug, Wal-Mart remained firm in its decision not to carry the product. The discount retailer also refused to budge when confronted with boycotts from feminist organizations. Roderick L. Mackenzie found that Preven was received more favorably by other major drugstore and discount chains. He told the *New York Times* that the drug was more favorably received by other drug retailers. "'I'd rather have every piece of business available in the world," he said, "but I'm realistic."[11] Other advocates for emergency contraception were not so resigned and decided to once again demand that the FDA take action on this issue.

OTCness and Emergency Contraception

In June 2000, the FDA scheduled a two-day hearing in response to numerous inquiries from pharmaceutical industry representatives and healthcare organizations about criteria for allowing a drug to be sold without a prescription. To be considered for OTC status, a drug had to treat conditions that a consumer could realistically self-diagnose without seeing a healthcare provider. The FDA also stipulated that labeling for the product be "true and understandable."[12]

At the hearing in June 2000, the FDA heard testimony from twenty-five speakers representing the drug industry, scientists, health insurance providers, drug-law experts, physicians groups, nonprofit organizations, and consumers. Many of those who spoke in favor of making certain categories of drugs available without prescription did so because it would allow patients to get these drugs more easily.[13]

The issue of access was especially important to advocates of emergency contraception. Kirsten Moore from the Reproductive Health Technologies Project argued that the calls to the organizations hotline and inquiries at the website indicated that many women had difficulty obtaining emergency contraceptive pills in a timely fashion. She gave an example of a woman trying to get an appointment with a healthcare provider on a weekend or succeeding in getting a prescription only to have a pharmacist refuse to fill it. The one concern of the RHTP and others in the women's health advocacy community was the issue of insurance reimbursement. Moore observed that women on a fixed or low-income might not be able to afford an OTC product if their health insurance did not reimburse them for it the way it did for prescription medications. "For this reason," Moore said, "we strongly encourage the FDA to consider maintaining dual status for ECPs" and allow the same products to be available both OTC and by prescription.[14]

Tara Shochet from the American Society for Emergency Contraception argued that there were no medical reasons to keep emergency contraceptive pills on prescription status. Women did not need help diagnosing the need for emergency contraception. "The doctor does not need to do a physical exam," she argued "and as with aspirin or decongestant, there's little harm done if a woman takes the pills when she doesn't actually need them." Therefore, "requiring a prescription for using emergency contraception is as foolish as requiring prescriptions for using fire extinguishers."[15]

Jack Stover from Gynetics claimed that over-the-counter status for Preven would not only enhance access but also increase awareness. Although the company had spent almost fifteen million dollars since the drug's launch in 1998, they had been able to only increase public awareness of emergency contraception to less than 10 percent of their target market. Gynetics had participated in independent studies and evaluations that showed OTC emergency contraception could be a one-hundred-million-dollar-a-year product with the proper level of advertising.[16]

Amy Allina from the National Women's Health Network explained why her organization supported making emergency contraception available without prescription but opposed doing the same for regular oral contraceptive pills. Like the FDA, the NWHN was "striving for consistency" in their position on which drugs should be available over the counter and shared the agency's concern that OTC products must have "a low incidence of adverse reactions" and "be intended for use in conditions that can readily be recognized by a consumer without the assistance of a clinician." For the NWHN, the logistical barriers to obtaining emergency contraception within the seventy-two-hour time period convinced them that prescription-only distribution of this product was unnecessary to ensure safe and effective use. The network supported OTC distribution of emergency contraceptive pills under the following conditions: first, there must be "appropriate label warnings to protect the health of women with contraindications to the use of emergency contraceptive pills." While there was no evidence of adverse reactions to the short dose of hormones contained in emergency contraceptive pills, the network believed that women with a history of blood clots should avoid using this method and that the label of an over-the-counter product had to contain "a clear and prominent warning explaining this precaution." The patient package insert should be in multiple languages and also employ techniques for women who could not read, such as pictorial representations. The package insert should warn women that the product did not offer protection against sexually transmitted infections. The network also wanted to preserve affordable access to emergency contraception. As long as this was a prescription product, it was covered by some insurance plans, but once the prescription requirement was removed, women would have to pay for these products out of pocket. Sometimes the switch to OTC status had led to an increase in the price of a drug. While it was impossible to predict what would happen with emergency contraception, the network argued that in order to prevent barriers based on cost, healthcare providers should continue to prescribe regular oral contraceptives for the Yuzpe method to women who could not afford an OTC product. Finally, the network and other advocates were concerned that making emergency contraceptive pills available without a prescription might make it less likely that women using this method in cases of sexual assault would receive counseling and medical follow-up. Therefore, the network supported efforts to make counseling and medical services accessible to sexual assault survivors who chose to pursue them and opposed policies that required survivors to obtain such services against their will.[17]

Although the NWHN favored making more OTC contraceptive options available to women, they opposed doing this for oral contraceptive pills for continuing, regular contraception. The network believed that prescription status for regular birth control pills was "necessary to maintain effective use of this method and to protect the health of women who choose to use it." Without the prescription requirement, there would be "no opportunity for a healthcare provider to screen out users who should not be taking oral contraceptives over the long-term." Furthermore, the opportunity for preventive healthcare and disease detection would be lost, a matter "of particular concern when it comes to women of color and low-income women who are already likely to have decreased access to such health services." Allina said the network would support a middle way between the current prescription status and OTC distribution, such as distribution by pharmacists from behind the counter as was done in some European countries.[18]

In addition, the network believed it was important that the consumers have access to "sufficient, accurate, and unbiased information" about a product to ensure they could make an informed decision about whether to take a drug. The network did not believe that a drug company would "make an unbiased judgment about what information should be conveyed to women or how best to convey it." Allina was especially concerned about direct-to-consumer advertisements and argued that these kinds of campaigns created by pharmaceutical companies were "not adequate information sources for consumers."[19]

The hearings ended with commentary by Susan Lavine Coleman from NCI Consulting, a firm that had worked with pharmaceutical companies on most of the OTC switches over the previous decade. She argued that the FDA's role in promoting the public health should extend beyond protecting the consumer from dangerous products, but should also include a proactive role in making products more readily available. As an example of the later role, she gave the recent history of emergency contraception. Because industry was not taking the initiative on this issue, the FDA stepped in and made the marketplace aware that the agency was receptive to an application for an emergency contraceptive product. Although big companies were still uninterested in taking such a risk, "the small ones stepped in and introduced products." Coleman suggested that the FDA continue to collaborate with industry by encouraging the development of more OTC products.[20] Although the purpose of this meeting was solely to solicit public comments on how to address future switches from prescription to nonprescription status, advocates for making emergency contraception available without prescription felt that the door had been opened for them to advance their cause.

Politics and Science at the FDA

In November 2000, Sharon Camp announced that Women's Capital Corporation (WCC) would apply to the FDA to approve making Plan B available over the counter. Despite testimony in favor of OTC status at the hearing in June, Gynetics decided not to take the same route for Preven. The company's founder, Roderick Mackenzie, raised doubts about whether eliminating the prescription requirement would raise women's awareness of emergency contraception, as Camp and other advocates of the OTC switch suggested. In addition, Mackenzie said that "going over the counter means that you have to use consumer advertising to get to women," and such advertising was more expensive than for prescription drugs. Finally, retail drugstores and supermarkets had "to see the product have enough volume to justify a space on the shelf."[21]

Camp soon began discussions with officials at the FDA about submitting a supplemental new drug application (SNDA) in order to remove the prescription requirement for Plan B. Meanwhile, other advocates decided to put direct pressure on the FDA to act quickly on making emergency contraception available over the counter. On February 14, 2001, the Center for Reproductive Law and Policy (CRLP) filed a citizen petition with the FDA on behalf of more than seventy organizations, including the American Public Health Association, the American Medical Women's Association, the Association of Reproductive Health Professionals, the National Asian Women's Health Organizations, the National Black Women's Health Project, the National Family Planning and Reproductive Health Association, the Planned Parenthood Federation of America, and the Reproductive Health Technologies Project. The petition requested that Preven and Plan B be made available without a prescription, arguing that under FDA regulations, any drug limited to prescription use should be exempted from prescription-dispensing requirements when the commissioner found such requirements were not necessary for the protection of the public health. The petitioners argued that emergency contraceptive pills met the above criteria in several ways. First, they were safe for self-medication because they were not toxic to the woman or to an embryo or fetus should the method fail; they had a low risk of abuse or overdose; and the side effects were well known and minor. Second, studies had shown that emergency contraceptive pills were effective when self-administered, and the decision whether to use these contraceptives was simple and relied on assessments that could be made independently by women themselves. Furthermore, the condition that was treated by emergency contraception—contraceptive failure or failure to use a contraceptive—was one that was "readily diagnosable by a woman." Fourth, the existing patient labeling for Preven and Plan B was "tailored to self-administration" in that it was "simple, clear, comprehensive, and easy to follow." Finally, switching emergency contraception to OTC status would "promote public health" because it would allow women to obtain this product in a timely fashion and "enable more women to prevent unwanted pregnancies." For these reasons, the petitioners requested that the FDA "explicitly authorize the use of a citizen petition to seek a switch from prescription to OTC status."[22]

In their affidavit supporting the petition, David Grimes and Elizabeth Raymond, obstetrician-gynecologists who had conducted extensive research on emergency contraception, argued that because of the "urgent need" to improve access and "the lack of any compelling reason to prohibit women from exercising control over this contraceptive method" family planning programs in the United States were already moving to "OTC-like" distribution methods for emergency contraceptive pills. For example, Planned Parenthood Federation of America had endorsed providing prescriptions for emergency contraceptive pills after a telephone consultation with a provider, as well as provision of pills in advance so that patients could keep them at home in case of future need. Grimes and Raymond argued that "these approaches are similar to over-the-counter distribution in that the patient is not examined before she takes the pills; and in the case of advance provision, she may not have had any screening or counseling by a medical professional for weeks, months, or even years before pill use." Planned Parenthood affiliate clinics and other reproductive health service clinics around the country had adopted these methods with no known problems. In conclusion, they argued that mandating a prescription for emergency contraception hurt women's health "by posing an unnecessary obstacle to the prompt, effective use of this important therapy." The prescription requirement also indirectly contributed to "the epidemic of unintended pregnancies and induced abortions in this country." These outcomes, they argued, were "both antithetical to the mission of the FDA and damaging to public health." They argued that the FDA should follow the Hippocratic principle of "first, do no harm" and drop the prescription requirement for emergency contraception.[23]

The FDA's Division of Reproductive and Urologic Drug Products immediately reviewed the citizen petition and on February 28 informed the petitioners that while the petition contained an affidavit and list of citations to medical literature from two medical experts in the field of emergency contraceptive research, the FDA's Division of OTC Drug Products (DOTCDP) required data from both a labeling comprehension study and actual use study of emergency contraceptive products before they would authorize a switch from prescription to over the counter. In a memo to the CLRP on April 12, 2001, the DOTCDP concluded that the citizen petition's contained insufficient data to support this switch. At the same time the FDA was communicating with WCC about the data needed to persuade the agency to allow Plan B to be sold over the counter. In April 2003, WCC submitted a SNDA seeking to switch the product from prescription-only to OTC status. On November 25, 2003, the FDA published a notice in the *Federal Register* announcing that a hearing for the SNDA for Plan

B would be held at a joint committee meeting of the Nonprescription Drugs Advisory Committee and the Advisory Committee for Reproductive Health Drugs on December 16, 2003.[24]

The announcement of the meeting prompted a flurry of activity from activists on both sides of the OTC debate. Over sixty medical associations—including the American College Health Association, the American Medical Association, the Society for Adolescent Medicine, and the American Academy of Pediatrics—wrote position papers expressing their support for the SNDA. These experts also testified at the joint committee meeting in December 2003. As Lisa Wynn argues in her analysis of the sexual archetypes that emerged in the discussions of the OTC switch for Plan B, scientists and physicians "framed their arguments in terms of the drug's safety and ability to reduce unplanned pregnancy and thus both pregnancy-related morbidity and abortion rates."[25] For example, Heather Boonstra from the Alan Guttmacher Institute argued, "Timely access to emergency contraception is one of the most promising avenues for lowering unintended pregnancy and reducing the need for abortion in the United States."[26]

These arguments were similar to the disease-based paradigm that has been used by proponents of the emergency contraception since the 1960s. As in the past, emergency contraception was presented as a "cure" for an "epidemic" of unwanted pregnancy. Even when consumer activists raised concerns about the safety of this method, physicians and population experts continued to believe that the dangers of contraceptive use were outweighed by the personal and social costs of contraceptive failure. Many opponents of the OTC change for ECP—especially pro-life health professionals—also cast their arguments in epidemiological terms. Opponents claimed that the failure rate of emergency contraception was higher than suggested by advocates and that making this available over the counter would actually contribute to the epidemic of teenage pregnancy. Opponents also claimed that increased availability of ECP would lead to soaring rates of sexually transmitted infections among American teenagers, even though label comprehension studies conducted for the SNDA indicated that women and girls clearly understood that Plan B did not prevent these diseases. These opponents also replicated anxieties about the uncontrolled sexuality of young women that formed the basis of some of the earliest studies of postcoital contraception during the 1960s. However, these opponents also believed that the cure for these public health crises was encouraging abstinence, not improving access to contraceptives and abortion. Retired internist Robert Carroll, for example, observed that over the previous ten years there had been a slow but steady increase in sexual abstinence accompanied by a correspondent decrease in abortions and teen pregnancies. Carroll concluded, "It is self-evident that over-the-counter availability of the morning after pill will lead to increased promiscuity and its attendant physical and psychological damage."[27]

As a counterpoint to these disease-based arguments for and against over-the-counter access, young women from various feminist organizations testified about their personal experiences with emergency contraception and the difficulties they had in obtaining the pills in a timely fashion. As in the congressional hearings on the Pill and other hormone drugs during the 1970s, women expressed their rights to bodily autonomy and informed medical decisions. However, rather than demanding protection from a dangerous product and from exploitation by medical researchers, these women emphasized their rights to choose contraceptive options without interference from doctors, pharmacists, or other health professionals.[28] Kelly Mangan, vice president of the University of Florida chapter of the National Organization for Women, declared: "Women should not be told when or under what circumstances we can control our bodies. Yet here I stand ironically before a panel many of whom are men having to ask for the right to control my body and direct my life." Erin Mahoney, co-chair of the National Organization for Women, New York State Reproductive Rights Task Force, described cases in which she was "lucky" enough to find a physician who was willing to write a prescription for ECP and other times when she was not so fortunate. "I shouldn't have to rely on luck to control my life," she exclaimed. "I shouldn't have to rely on a doctor for a drug that is safe and effective within the first 24 hours after sex." Linda Freeman, co-chair of the NOW New York State Reproductive Rights Task Force, addressed concerns that teenage and young adult women would misuse or abuse ECP: "Please do not insult our intelligence nor belittle us. We as women are capable of following directions." Moreover, "we as women should and must be allowed to make reproductive decisions for ourselves without interference from others, without judgment from others, and without the need for someone else' approval."[29]

At the end of the hearing, the joint advisory committee voted in favor of switching Plan B to nonprescription status. Supporters of the SNDA were delighted but also surprised that they had prevailed given the generally unfavorable environment for reproductive choice under the George W. Bush administration. James Trussell, a member of the panel who voted for the recommendation, told the *New York Times,* "It's hard to believe it actually happened." Kirsten Moore from the RHTP told the same reporter, "I guess I just didn't have a lot of faith that people would let the facts speak for themselves."[30]

This guarded optimism would soon turn to disappointment: on May 6, 2004, Dr. Steven Galson, then acting director of the FDA's Center for Drug Evaluation and Research, rejected the recommendation of the joint advisory committee and issued a non-approvable letter to Barr Laboratories (which had purchased the patent rights to Plan B from WCC). Galson argued that Barr had "not provided adequate data to support a conclusion that Plan B® can be used safely by young adolescent women for emergency contraception without the professional supervision of a practitioner licensed by law to administer the drug." Galson told Barr that it had to either submit data demonstrating that the product could be used safely by women under seventeen years of age without professional supervision by a licensed practitioner or provide an alternate proposal to allow for marketing of Plan B as a prescription-only product for women under seventeen and as an OTC product for women aged seventeen and older.[31] Galson's suggestion was the first time in its history that the FDA had advised that a drug be assigned to a prescription status based on age.[32]

Because Galson and the four joint advisory committee members who had voted against the OTC switch were political appointees of President George W. Bush, advocates of nonprescription status for emergency contraception declared that these FDA officials were allowing the president's anti-choice agenda to override their responsibility to be unbiased guardians of the public health. "Politics trumps science at the U.S. Food and Drug Administration," declared David Grimes in the journal *Obstetrics and Gynecology,* coining a catch phrase that was widely repeated in other media reports of the FDA decision. Barr submitted a revised application on July 22, 2004, but the FDA delayed ruling on it for over two years.[33] Meanwhile, some feminist activists were running out of patience and decided to take more direct action to promote the cause of OTC emergency contraception.

The Morning-After Pill Conspiracy

While the FDA was considering Barr's SNDA for Plan B, the docket for the citizen petition filed by CRLP remained open, and FDA continued to receive public comments from both proponents and opponents of nonprescription status for emergency contraception. After several requests from petitioners that the agency act on the citizen petition, and following the statutory deadline for the FDA to rule on the revised application, on January 21, 2005, the CRLP (now renamed the Center for Reproductive Rights or CRR) filed a lawsuit in the U.S. District Court for the Eastern District of New York on behalf of the Association of Reproductive Health Professionals (ARHP), National Latina Institute for

Reproductive Health, and individuals from a grassroots advocacy group called the Morning-After Pill Conspiracy (MAPC).[34]

The lead plaintiff in the case, Annie Tummino, worked for Realbirth, a childbirth education and postpartum support center in New York City, and was chair of the Women's Liberation Birth Control Project. Tummino formed the MAPC in 2004 out of a coalition of feminist organizations dedicated to making emergency contraception available without prescription for all women regardless of age. Several founding members of the MAPC had testified at the joint advisory committee meeting on the OTC switch for Plan B. Tummino said MAPC was inspired by the grassroots activism of the women's liberation movement of the 1960s and 1970s: "We speak out and engage in civil disobedience. Our goal is to send the message that women are the experts on our bodies and lives."[35] The group's name was "a tongue-in-cheek reference to the fact that under such restrictive conditions many women obtained these pills from a friend, thus conspiring to break the law just to get a safe form of birth control." Because getting a prescription from a doctor and filling it within the time frame was "virtually impossible for most women," many women sought out friends "who worked in health clinics to gain access and to stockpile packages for friends."[36]

In addition to filing the lawsuit, the MAPC used a variety of direct-action techniques to protest the FDA's and the Bush administration's stance on emergency contraception. They held consciousness-raising sessions and speak-outs in major cities and committed various acts of civil disobedience, including passing along emergency contraceptive kits to women without a prescription. Most emblematic of their ties to second-wave feminist organizing were their actions at the March for Women's Lives in Washington, D.C., on April 25, 2004. The group held a mini-rally where a dozen women "testified about rushing around trying to get the Morning-After Pill after a condom broke during sex, about the prohibitive costs associated with a doctor's visit, and about the tragicomic idea that anyone can get a doctor's appointment in twenty-four hours, especially starting on a Friday or Saturday night." In defiance of "unjust" prescription laws, the group flung boxes of Plan B into the crowd. They also invited spectators "to join them in signing the Morning-After Pill Conspiracy pledge to defy the prescription requirement (and break the law) by giving a friend the Morning-After Pill whenever she needs it." A group of physicians from the Association of Reproductive Health Professionals' Reproductive Health Access Project contributed to this display of feminist direct action by freely writing prescriptions for emergency contraception for any woman who requested one. According to MAPC member Jenny Brown, these doctors "were illustrating a point which was repeated over and over in the FDA's advisory hearings—no physical evaluation or instruction from medical professionals is needed to safely and effectively use this medication." Members of MAPC declared they "were proud to follow in the footsteps of feminists like Margaret Sanger, who passed out information on birth control when it was illegal to do so, and suffragists who were arrested for voting, to showcase how unjust the laws were."[37]

In June 2004, the MAPC sent a letter to Galison condemning the agency's "sexist decision" to reject Barr's application for over-the-counter sales of Plan B. The MAPC declared that by ignoring the opinion of its own advisory committees, the FDA had "put politics over science by towing the anti-birth control line of President Bush and other conservative extremists. You, and the extremists to whom you answer, have contributed to making the U.S. more backward on birth control than 38 other countries that do not require a prescription for the Morning-After Pill (MAP)." Attached to the letter was a petition with over fifteen hundred signatures of women who pledged "to break the law by giving out our prescription-only morning after pills to friends who need them." The group observed that "women routinely resort to this 'criminal' behavior due to the current inaccessibility of MAP, and we're proudly going public with our actions to show how ridiculous and unjust the prescription requirement truly is."[38] Like the feminist activists who protested against the abuse of women subjects during the 1970s, MAPC members held a sit-in at FDA headquarters in January of 2005, where nine of their members were arrested for blocking access to the FDA, "just like they were blocking women's access to birth control."[39]

By filing the lawsuit against, Tummino hoped to show that the FDA had not been following normal procedures and had held Barr's SNDA "to a much higher standard than any other application."[40] Tummino and the other plaintiffs charged that the FDA's suggestion that Barr file a dual prescription/nonprescription application for Plan B violated their rights and the rights of women who needed Plan B to privacy and equal protection under the Fifth Amendment. Plaintiffs also charged the agency with "failure to follow medical science in their decisions on the MAP." The lawsuit sought the removal of the age restriction and behind-the-counter status for Plan B.[41] In a position paper, MAPC member Brown argued that the age restriction had bad effects for all women, not just those under sixteen: "If we allow them to pit us against each other by age we will lose the chance to get what we really want, the Morning After Pill over the counter for all women." The organization would not "accept the insult that young women are irresponsible when we try to obtain after-sex birth control. That is us taking responsibility."[42]

Feminists on Capitol Hill aided the efforts of the MAPC to force the FDA to cease stalling on the Plan B decision. After President Bush nominated Lester Crawford as commissioner of the FDA, Senators Patty Murray (D-WA) and Hillary Rodham Clinton (D-NY) announced in April 2005 that they would block a vote on Crawford's confirmation until the FDA ruled on Barr's SNDA. Senators Murray and Clinton released their hold in Crawford's nomination after Health and Human Services secretary Michael Leavitt promised he would make sure that the FDA would rule on the Plan B application by September 1. After being confirmed as FDA commissioner on July 18, Crawford announced that rather than rendering a final decision Barr's SNDA, the FDA would invite public comment on the "novel regulatory issues" that would be raised should the agency take the unprecedented step of approving dual packaging for the same drug. Susan Wood, director of the FDA Office of Women's Health, resigned in protest against Crawford's decision, stating that she could no longer work at an agency where "scientific evidence and clinical evidence, fully evaluated and recommended for approval for the professional staff here, has been overruled." Wood added that morale among FDA staff was low following Crawford's actions, as they worried that this would "severely damage the agency's credibility." Senators Murray and Clinton stated that Wood's resignation was another casualty of the Bush administration's "suppressing science when it doesn't fit their political agenda."[43]

In the wake of public outcry following Wood's resignation, Commissioner Crawford also resigned abruptly for undisclosed reasons, and President Bush named Andrew von Eschenbach, a family friend and head of the National Cancer Institute, as acting commissioner. The image of the FDA was further tarnished by a report from the Government Accountability Office (GAO) issued in November 2005. The report found that four aspects of the agency's review of the Plan B over-the-counter switch application were unusual. First, although the directors of the Offices of Drug Evaluation supported the advisory committee's recommendation on the OTC switch, they were pressured by higher-level management to draft a non-approval letter, which the directors refused to sign. Second, the GAO report found that this involvement by high-level management was much greater than was usually the case for OTC applications. Third, FDA officials had conflicting accounts about when the decision to not approve Plan B was made. Finally, the decision of CDER acting director Steven Galison was "novel and did not follow FDA's traditional practices" in that the agency had never before considered differences in cognitive development between adolescents and adults when making a ruling on an OTC switch. The GAO report also observed that the decision on Plan B was the only prescription-to-over-the-counter decision made between 1994 and 2004 in which the CDER director overruled the recommendations of a joint advisory committee.[44]

The FDA continued to delay action on the Plan B over-the-counter decision despite threats from Senators Clinton and Murray that they would stall von Eschenbach's confirmation as permanent commissioner of the FDA. In June 2006, the FDA formally denied the citizen petition, again citing lack of adequate data on safe use by adolescent girls. Finally, on August 23, 2006, the agency approved the sale of Plan B without prescription, but only to those aged eighteen and over. To ensure enforcement of the age restriction, the drug could only be sold in pharmacies or other facilities staffed by a healthcare professional and kept behind the counter so that it could be dispensed only to those who could show proof of age.

Senators Murray and Clinton dropped their hold on von Eschenbach's confirmation, but Tummino and her fellow plaintiffs did not drop their lawsuit against the FDA. Following the agency's rejection of the citizen petition filed by CRR, the lead attorney in the case, Simon Heller, declared: "The FDA's rejection of our citizen's petition in the midst of this lawsuit simply confirms what we have believed all along. The FDA, in the thrall of the Bush administration's anti-science agenda, has put aside its mission to promote public health in favor of depriving women of easier access to this important drug."[45] The CRR attorneys requested depositions from key FDA officials related to the case, including former commissioners Lester Crawford and Mark McClellan, Deputy Commissioner Janet Woodcock, former Office of Women's Health director Susan Wood, and the director of the Center for Drug Evaluation and Research, Steven Galson. The judge in the case also allowed the plaintiffs to subpoena White House documents for the lawsuit, citing "strong showing of bad faith" as grounds for granting further discovery in the case. On March 23, 2009, the U.S. District Court for the Eastern District of New York ruled that the FDA "had put politics before women's health" when it decided to limit over-the-counter access to the emergency contraceptive Plan B to women over age eighteen. The court ordered the agency to reconsider its decision and to act within thirty days to extend nonprescription status to seventeen-year-olds.[46]

The Morning-After Pill Conspiracy was jubilant: on their website, they declared this decision was "a huge victory for women's liberation." It also demonstrated the power of feminist organizing: "All along, feminists have accused the FDA of toeing the anti-birth control line of the Bush Administration in their decision making on the Morning-After Pill." By taking to the streets and the courts, the MAPC and other feminist health organizations had convinced the court that the FDA had acted arbitrarily in denying OTC access to emergency contraception for girls under eighteen.[47] In April 2009, the FDA said it would follow the court's orders and allow Barr to make its product available to seventeen-year-olds without a prescription. Cécile Richards, president of Planned Parenthood Federation of America, said this announcement was "a strong statement to American women that their health comes before politics."[48] In August 2009, the FDA approved Watson Labs' Next Choice, the first generic version of Plan B, for OTC sales to consumers aged seventeen and older. Yet, other nonprescription emergency contraceptive products were still restricted to those eighteen and older. The FDA claimed that it needed applications from each manufacturer in order to comply with the court ruling. The CCR disagreed and on November 16, 2010, filed a motion for contempt of court against the FDA for patently ignoring the court's order and continuing its "administrative stall" on the citizen's petition filed in 2000. The CRR argued that the agency's disregard of the court's "clear and lawful order" harmed women under the age of eighteen whose access to Plan B was hindered by the arbitrary age restrictions imposed by the FDA. The CRR argued that the agency had now "had ample time, sufficient information, and countless opportunities to rule upon the petition." The FDA had not only "failed to do so," but also "asserted that it is not taking any affirmative steps to rule on it and has no plans to do so in the near future." Because the FDA had failed to comply with the court's order in a timely and reasonable manner, the plaintiffs respectfully requested "that the Court find the FDA in contempt, direct the FDA to issue a decision on the Citizen Petition within forty-five days of the contempt finding, and order any other relief that the Court deems fair and appropriate."[49] The FDA has yet to act on this motion.

The battle for OTC emergency contraception is an example of how feminist grassroots activism on emergency contraception has helped redefine the meaning of the prescription in the early twenty-first century. The civil disobedience of the MAPC against the "injustice" of the prescription as a barrier for emergency contraception is one way in which feminist health activists continue to assert women's rights to control their own bodies in opposition to institutions of medical authority. The participation of healthcare professionals in this activism suggests that at least in the case of emergency contraception, the threat to professional authority posed by the erosion of the prescription is outweighed by the public health goal of preventing unwanted pregnancy.

The appointment of a more progressive leadership to the FDA by President Barack Obama made emergency contraception advocates hopeful that the agency would take a more objective stance on this birth control technology. Reproductive rights activists were especially encouraged by the agency's approval of a new emergency contraceptive—ulipristal acetate (trade name ellaOne) in August 13, 2010. This drug was considered an improvement over the levonorgestral regime because it was effective up to five days after unprotected sex. During the FDA's deliberations, the NWHN feared a repeat of the agency's "shameful history" of the Plan B approval process. In their testimony before the FDA Reproductive Health Drugs Advisory Committee, the NWHN noted that the agency had "lost considerable credibility in the eyes of women, clinicians, and regulators" during the Plan B proceedings "because its leadership at the time was seen to override the conclusions and recommendations of scientific staff and expert advisors in order to satisfy political aims." The network "urged the FDA not to dig itself a deeper hole by pursuing a similar path" with the ellaOne application. The NWHN also aggressively fought anti-abortion groups who appropriated the language of safety in order to derail the ellaOne approval. Amy Allina wrote, "We used our credibility as long-time drug safety advocates" to point out that hundreds of drugs came before FDA each year, yet these same critics did not raise similar concerns about these applications "because their goal is not drug safety, but rather to hamper women's access to another contraceptive option." The advisory committee agreed with NWHN and other advocates who testified and voted against putting any distribution restrictions on ellaOne. In marked contrast to the Plan B episode, the FDA leadership approved the advisory committee's recommendation. The network commended the FDA "for a thorough, science-based review of ulipristal acetate" and an approval process that "demonstrated that the agency is no longer allowing a political agenda to override its decision-making capacity." The NWHN hoped that the FDA would "complete the job by eliminating the medically unjustified age restriction on over-the-counter distribution" of Plan B and other levonorgestral emergency contraceptives, which continued "to undermine public trust in the agency."[50] Whether the agency will fulfill these expectations remains to be seen.

Conclusion

In an editorial for the journal *Contraception* in 2009, Francine Coeytaux, Elisa Wells, and Elizabeth Westley summarized the success of a twenty-year battle by women's health advocates to bring emergency contraception "from secret to shelf." Accomplishments included the creation of dedicated products, an increase in women's awareness and use of this contraceptive method, and increased access through over-the-counter sales for women seventeen and older. Yet, despite this progress, the authors observed that advocates of emergency contraception had "encountered a curve ball that has us circling back where we started." Analyses of the impact of growing availability of emergency contraception indicated that this technology had not fulfilled the promise of substantially reducing unwanted pregnancy on the population level. Rather than blaming this on user error, the editorial suggested that the population model aimed at reducing the epidemic of unwanted pregnancies and abortions was outdated and insulting to women. They and other reproductive health professionals needed to acknowledge "that individual women have a right to use the contraceptive method that best suits them, not the one that best contributes to overall demographic indicators." The editorial observed that "women's health advocates have fought long and hard to make 'choice,' not demographic indicators, the foundation of reproductive health services." Emergency contraception was an excellent example of expanding choice, not only because it gave women a second chance to prevent pregnancy, but also because women could obtain this drug themselves with minimal intervention by the medical profession. The editorial urged other reproductive health and donor communities to not give up on emergency contraception just because it was not proving to be as effective on a population level as originally expected. Instead, professionals in the field should protect women's access to this contraceptive choice so they could "decide for themselves how EC [emergency contraception] fits into their plans to avoid an unintended pregnancy."[1]

The editorial correctly observed that emergency contraception had come "full circle" in the sense that it had failed to fulfill the promise of "curing" the "disease" of unwanted pregnancy. It has not even filled the hopes of feminist activists that all women could access this product without any interference from health professionals. Emergency contraceptives are not literally available over the counter but are kept behind the counter, and customers must show identification proving they are old enough to purchase them. This is not the only OTC drug product sold this way. A number of states have recently passed laws or regulations requiring cold medicines containing the decongestant pseudoephedrine to be placed behind the pharmacy counter to prevent the bulk purchase of the drug to manufacture crystal methamphetamine. These developments have in effect created a third class of drugs whose restricted market is no longer defined in terms of the prescription but by the nature of the "counter." This means that pharmacists have replaced physicians and nurse practitioners as the gatekeepers for certain classes of drugs. It also has allowed some pharmacists to create new barriers to medication access by asserting that they have a right to conscientiously refuse to sell emergency contraception on religious grounds.[2]

Yet, by endorsing the language of choice and women's rights used by feminist health activists, the editorial illustrated how the attitudes of some reproductive health professionals had changed considerably over the past half century. During the 1960s, the "morning-after pill" was touted as a solution to the worldwide population crisis and the "epidemic" of unwed pregnancy in the United States. This shift in perspective reflected the professionalization of the women's health movement. Since the 1970s, feminist health activists had gradually become insiders in reproductive health by earning professional credentials, which gave them the ability to reform organized medicine and healthcare policy from within. Although some of their contemporaries accused these newly minted professionals of "selling-out," the corresponding radical-ization of the medical establishment had a profound affect on reproductive healthcare for women.

This transformation led health professionals to reevaluate the older disease-based argument that drove innovation in contraceptive technology. An emphasis on rights also gave advocates a way to prevent opponents from co-opting messages about risk and safety used by earlier feminist critics of hormonal contraception. In her testimony at the over-the-counter hearings for Plan B, thirty-five-year-old Amanda Leader, co-chair of Red Stockings Allies and Veterans in New York City, remarked, "Even with my activist experience with the pill, I still didn't know that its side effects had been wildly exaggerated," especially by pro-life activists who argued against nonprescription status. "I hadn't heard women talk about taking it like we're doing here today," she said. "This is why women need to speak out from our own experiences with the morning after pill and birth control to find out what's really going on."[3]

Other historians have argued that "body knowledge" was central to the women's health activism of second-wave feminism and that this feminist framework was abandoned as the women's health movement adopted the professional credentials and scientific language of the healthcare establishment.[4] I argue that rather than being a departure from second-wave feminist strategies that were based on knowledge of the biological body, recent activism on emergency contraception demonstrates how women have continued to use personal histories of their bodies to transform reproductive health research and healthcare policy. Since the early 1990s, emergency contraception has served as a bridge issue that has brought together former adversaries, including feminist health organizations, population and family planning people, and groups representing women of color, who were the main targets of attempts to control the population crisis in the United States. In order to bring more radical groups onboard, mainstream population organizations and reproductive health professionals had to overcome much bad faith generated by sexism in the medical profession and the often coercive policies of the population movement.

A narrow focus on purely technological solutions to the complex social problem of pregnancy prevention could dissolve this fragile alliance. Therefore, as experts and activists continue to strategize on how to make emergency contraception and other birth control products available to all women, it is imperative that the language of rights and reproductive choice remain at the forefront of these deliberations.

In addition, the recent battle for OTC emergency contraception provides a template for those interested in expanding women's contraceptive options in the twenty-first century. This case shows that removing a drug out from behind the aegis of the prescription does not make it immediately accessible to all who might benefit from it. Nonetheless, many of the individuals involved in achieving the OTC status for Plan B are eager to extend this precedent to the sphere of regular oral contraceptives. In 2004, a number of these parties formed the Oral Contraceptives Over-the-Counter Working Group "to explore the potential of over-the-counter access to oral contraceptives to reduce disparities in reproductive healthcare access and outcomes, and to increase opportunities for women to access a safe, effective method of contraception, free of unnecessary control, as part of a healthy sexual and reproductive life."[5] In November 2007, the FDA held a public meeting on behind the counter (BTC) availability of certain drugs, at which the NWHN's Amy Allina argued that the prescription was a significant barrier to access and compliance since some women discontinued pill use because they could not schedule an appointment with a healthcare provider before the prescription ran out. If the creation of a BTC class of drugs were "well executed," she argued, then this could address some of these problems with access and compliance. On the other hand, she said, a "poorly-executed BTC system could make existing problems worse or even create new barriers for women" if health insurance did not cover BTC contraceptives.[6]

The most recent health reform legislation does not look promising in this regard: the health insurance plans will not cover nonprescription drugs, and the new law will prohibit the use of flexible spending accounts for OTC drugs as well. The congressional elections of November 2010 created a Republican majority in the House of Representatives, which threatens to repeal the health reform law completely. The rise of the feminist health movement and other consumer empowerment initiatives over the past several decades has had uneven consequences. Although they have weakened the boundary between patients and the healthcare professionals, they have thus far been unable to resolve the economic inequalities in the United States that continue to pose an insurmountable barrier to those unable to afford the products of this self-care revolution.

Notes

Introduction

1. Robert A. Hatcher, James Trussell, Felicia Stewart, et al., *Emergency Contraception: The Nation's Best-Kept Secret* (Decataur, GA: Bridging the Gap Communications, 1995); Barbara Pillsbury, Francine Coeytaux, and Andrea Johnson, *From Secret to Shelf: How Collaboration Is Bringing Emergency Contraception to Women* (Los Angeles: Pacific Institute for Women's Health, 1999).
2. For more information on current methods of emergency contraception, see the Emergency Contraception website, http://ec.princeton.edu/ (accessed June 2, 2009).
3. Margaret Marsh and Wanda Ronner, *The Fertility Doctor: John Rock and the Reproductive Revolution* (Baltimore: Johns Hopkins University Press, 2008).
4. For more on the development of DES and other synthetic estrogens, see Elizabeth Siegel Watkins, *The Estrogen Elixir: A History of Hormone Replacement Therapy in America* (Baltimore: Johns Hopkins University Press, 2007), 10–31.
5. Barbara Seaman and Gideon Seaman, *Women and the Crisis in Sex Hormones* (New York: Rawson Associates Publishers, 1977).
6. For example, see Barbara Ehrenreich and Deidre English, *For Her Own Good: 150 Years of the Experts' Advice to Women* (New York: Anchor Press, 1978).
7. Elizabeth Watkins, *On the Pill: A Social History of Oral Contraceptives, 1950–1970* (Baltimore: Johns Hopkins University Press, 1998); Lara Marks, *Sexual Chemistry: A History of the Pill* (New Haven: Yale University Press, 2001); Andrea Tone, *Devices and Desires: A History of Contraceptives in America* (New York: Hill and Wang, 2001); and Johanna Schoen, *Choice and Coercion: Birth Control, Sterilization, and Abortion in Public Health and Welfare* (Chapel Hill: University of North Carolina Press, 2005).
8. Adele Clarke and Theresa Montini, "The Many Faces of RU486: Tales of Situated Knowledges and Technological Contestations," *Science, Technology, and Human Values* 18 (1993): 42.
9. Schoen, *Choice and Coercion*, 22–23.
10. Wendy Kline, *Bodies of Knowledge: Sexuality, Reproduction, and Women's Health in the Second Wave* (Chicago: University of Chicago Press, 2010); Susan Reverby, "Thinking through the Body and the Body Politic: Feminism, History, and Health-Care Policy in the United States," in *Women, Health, and Nation: Canada and the United States since 1945,* edited by Georgina Feldberg, Molly Ladd-Taylor, Alison Li, and Kathryn McPherson (Montreal: McGill-Queen's University Press, 2003), 404–420.

Chapter 1 — A Second Revolution in Birth Control

1. Lawrence Lader, "Three Men Who Made a Revolution," *New York Times,* April 10, 1966, 58.
2. Lara Marks, "Parenting the Pill: Early Testing of the Contraceptive Pill," in *Bodies*

of Technology: Women's Involvement with Reproductive Medicine, edited by Ann Rudinow Saetnan, Nelly Oudshoorn, and Marta Kirejczyk (Columbus: Ohio State University Press, 2000), 146.

3. Ellen Chesler, *Woman of Valor: Margaret Sanger and the Birth Control Movement in America* (New York: Simon and Schuster, 1992); R. Christian Johnson, "Feminism, Philanthropy, and Science in the Development of the Oral Contraceptive Pill," *Pharmacy in History* 19, no. 2 (1977): 63–78.

4. For more on the history of oral contraceptives, see Lara Marks, *Sexual Chemistry: A History of the Pill* (New Haven: Yale University Press, 2001); Andrea Tone, *Devices and Desires: A History of Contraceptives in America* (New York: Hill and Wang, 2001); Elizabeth Watkins, *On the Pill: A Social History of Oral Contraceptives, 1950–1970* (Baltimore: Johns Hopkins University Press, 1998); Leon Speroff, *A Good Man, Gregory Pincus: The Man, His Story, the Birth Control Pill* (Portland, OR: Arnica Publishing, 2009); and Elaine Tyler May, *American and the Pill: A History of Promise, Peril, and Liberation* (New York: Basic Books, 2010).

5. Watkins, *On the Pill,* 80–81.

6. Elizabeth Siegel Watkins, "From Breakthrough to Bust: The Brief Life of Norplant, the Contraceptive Implant," *Journal of Women's History* 22 (2010): 88–111.

7. Carrie Eisert, "Psychiatry, Gynecology, and the Effort to Understand Emotional Reactions to Oral Contraception," paper presented at the annual meeting of the American Association for the History of Medicine, Cleveland, Ohio, April 30, 2009; Patricia Peck Gossel, "Packaging the Pill," in *Manifesting Medicine: Bodies and Machines,* edited by Robert Bud, Bernard S. Finn, and Helmuth Trischler (Amsterdam, the Netherlands: Harwood Academic, 1999), 105–122.

8. Johanna Schoen, *Choice and Coercion: Birth Control, Sterilization, and Abortion in Public Health and Welfare* (Chapel Hill: University of North Carolina Press, 2005).

9. A. S. Parkes and C. W. Bellerby, "The Effects of the Injection of Oestrus-Producing Hormone during Pregnancy," *Journal of Physiology* 62 (1926): 145–155.

10. H. O. Burdick and G. Pincus, "The Effect of Oestrin Injections upon the Developing Ova of Mice and Rabbits," *American Journal of Physiology* 11 (1935): 201–208.

11. A. S. Parkes, E. C. Dodds, and R. L. Noble, "Interruption of Early Pregnancy by Means of Orally Active Oestrogens," *British Medical Journal* (1938):557–559.

12. Johnson, "Feminism, Philanthropy, and Science," 68–69; Speroff, *A Good Man,* 85–92.

13. For more on the history of the Worcester Foundation for Experimental Biology, see Speroff, *A Good Man,* 97–130; Tone, *Devices and Desires,* 209–213; and Hudson Hoagland, *The Road to Yesterday* (Worcester, MA: privately printed, 1974), 75–104.

14. Min Chueh Chang, "Mammalian Sperm, Eggs, and Control of Fertility," *Perspectives in Biology and Medicine* 11/3 (1968): 376–378.

15. Elaine Tyler May, *Barren in the Promised Land: Childless Americans and the Pursuit of Happiness* (New York: Basic Books, 1997).

16. Margaret Marsh and Wanda Ronner, *The Fertility Doctor: John Rock and the Reproductive Revolution* (Baltimore: Johns Hopkins University Press, 2008).

17. Quoted in Johnson, "Feminism, Philanthropy, and Science," 68.

18. Marks, *Sexual Chemistry,* 50–59, 96–97; Watkins, *On the Pill,* 21–25; Tone, *Devices and Desires,* 216–219.

19. Quote in Laura Briggs, *Reproducing Empire: Race, Sex, Science, and U.S. Imperialism in Puerto Rico* (Berkeley: University of California Press, 2002), 132–133. See

also Annette B. Ramirez and Conrad Seipp, *Colonialism, Catholicism, and Contraception: A History of Birth Control in Puerto Rico* (Chapel Hill: North Carolina Press, 1983); Martha C. Ward, *Poor Women, Powerful Men: America's Great Experiment on Family Planning* (Boulder, CO: Westview Press, 1986).

20. For more on the impact of the Nuremberg Code on American research involving human subjects, see David J. Rothman, *Strangers at the Bedside* (New York: Basic Books, 1991), 68–69. For more on the history of the Tuskegee study, see James H. Jones, *Bad Blood: The Tuskegee Syphilis Experiment* (New York: Free Press, 1981); and Susan M. Reverby, *Examining Tuskegee: The Infamous Syphilis Study and Its Legacy* (Chapel Hill: University of North Carolina Press, 2009).

21. Marks, *Sexual Chemistry,* 89–115; Watkins, *On the Pill,* 31–32; Tone, *Devices and Desires,* 225–231.

22. Watkin, *On the Pill,* 34–42; Tone, *Devices and Desires,* 234–236.

23. Margaret Marsh and Wanda Ronner, *The Fertility Doctor: John Rock and the Reproductive Revolution* (Baltimore: Johns Hopkins University Press, 2008).

24. Chang, "Mammalian Sperm," 382.

25. Johnson, "Feminism, Philanthropy, and Science," 63–64.

26. Linda Gordon shows that Sanger privately expressed ambivalence about surrendering control of the birth control movement to medical professionals. Linda Gordon, *The Moral Property of Women: A History of Birth Control Politics in America* (Chicago: University of Illinois Press, 2002).

27. Gwen Kay, *Dying to Be Beautiful: The Fight for Safe Cosmetics* (Columbus: Ohio State University Press, 2005), 3–5.

28. Margaret Sanger, "Editorial," *Birth Control Review* 5 (March 1921): 3–4, in the document project, "How Did the Debate between Margaret Sanger and Mary Ware Dennett Shape the Movement to Legalize Birth Control, 1915–1924?" by Melissa Doak and Rachel Brugger (Alexandria, VA: Alexander Street Press, 2000), Women and Social Movements database, alexander-street.com/products/wasm.htm (subscription only).

29. Durham-Humphrey Amendment, 503; 21 U.S.C.353

30. *Griswold v. Connecticut,* 381 U.S. 479 (1965). For more on the evolution of the concept of the right of privacy in American jurisprudence, see David J. Garrow, *Liberty and Sexuality: The Right to Privacy and the Making of Roe v. Wade* (Berkeley: University of California Press, 1998); and John W. Johnson, *Griswold v. Connecticut: Birth Control and the Constitutional Right of Privacy* (Lawrence: University of Kansas Press, 2005).

31. Harriet F. Pilpel and Nancy F. Wechsler, "Birth Control, Teenagers, and the Law," *Family Planning Perspectives* 1, no. 1 (Spring 1969): 29–35.

32. Gloria Steinem, "The Moral Disarmament of Betty Coed," *Esquire* 58 (September 1962), 97, 153–157.

33. Art Goldberg, "The Perils of the Pill," *Ramparts* 7 (May 1969): 45.

34. Carrie Eisert, "The Psychiatry of Birth Control Pill Acceptance, 1967–1973," paper presented at the annual meeting of the History of Science Society, Arlington, VA, November 2007.

35. Quoted in Watkins, *On the Pill,* 42.

36. For more on the history of FDA regulations, see Philip J. Hilts, *Protecting America's Health: The FDA, Business, and One Hundred Years of Regulation* (New York: Alfred A. Knopf, 2003). The critical role of women's organizations in the creation of drug regulations is described by Kay, *Dying to Be Beautiful.*

37. Tone, *Devices and Desires,* 243–244.

38. Watkins, *On the Pill,* 100.
39. Lawrence Lader, "Why Birth Control Fails," *McCall's* 97, no. 10 (1969): 163.
40. Carrie Eisert, "Psychiatry, Gynecology, and the Effort to Understand Emotion Reactions to Oral Contraception," paper presented at the annual meeting of the American Association for the History of Medicine, Cleveland, Ohio, April 23–26, 2009.
41. Barbara Seaman, "Why Did Birth Control Fail for Me?" *Ladies' Home Journal* 82 (1965): 166–167.
42. Jael Silliman, Marlene Gerber Fried, Loretta Ross, and Elena R. Gutiérrez, *Undivided Rights: Women of Color Organize for Reproductive Justice* (Cambridge, MA: South End Press, 2004), 54–55.
43. M. C. Chang, "Degeneration of Ova in the Rat and Rabbit Following Oral Administration of 1-(P-2-Diethylaminoethoxyphenyl)-1-Phenyl-2-P-Anisylethanol," *Endocrinology* 65, no. 2 (1959): 339–342; Chang and M. J. Harper, "Effects of Ethinyl Estradiol on Egg Transport and Development in the Rabbit," *Endocrinology* 78, no. 4 (1966): 860–872; Chang, "Effects of Oral Administration of Medroxyprogesterone Acetate and Ethinyl Estradiol on the Transportation and Development of Rabbit Eggs," *Endocrinology* 79, no. 5 (1966): 939–948; Chang, "Effects of Progesterone and Related Compounds on Fertilization, Transportation, and Development of Rabbit Eggs," *Endocrinology* 81, no. 6 (1967): 1251–1260.
44. Chang, "Mammalian Sperm," 381–382.
45. Chang, quoted in Lader, "Three Men Who Made a Revolution," 58.
46. Ibid., 55.
47. "Dr. Pincus, Developer of Birth-Control Pill, Dies," *New York Times,* August 23, 1967, 45; Alfonso A. Narvaez, "M. C. Chang, Scientist, Dies at 82: A Developer of Birth-Control Pill," *New York Times,* June 7, 1991, B6.
48. John McLean Morris, "Agents Affecting the Development of the Fertilized Ovum," *Transactions of the New England Obstetrical and Gynecological Society* 18 (1964): 57; Alton Blakeslee, "Sex Problem Discussed by Surgeons," *New York Times,* October 16, 1962, 27.
49. Morris, "Agents Affecting the Development," 57.
50. John McLean Morris and Gertrude van Wagenen, "Post-coital Oral Contraception," *Proceedings of the Eighth International Conference of the International Planned Parenthood Federation, Santiago, Chile* (IPPF, 1967), 256.
51. "New Pill Developed at Yale Advances Birth Control Study," *Hartford Courant,* May 1, 1966, 3A; Jane Brody, "Human Tests Considered," *New York Times,* May 1, 1966, 1.
52. Roberta Apfel and Susan M. Fisher, *To Do No Harm: DES and the Dilemmas of Modern Medicine* (New Haven: Yale University Press, 1984), 12–14.
53. Elizabeth Siegel Watkins, *The Estrogen Elixir: A History of Hormone Replacement Therapy in America* (Baltimore: Johns Hopkins University Press, 2007), 28–29; Apfel and Fisher, *To Do No Harm,* 16–20.
54. "Estrogens' Double Life," *Science News* 92 (1967): 343.

Chapter 2 — Courageous Volunteers

1. John McLean Morris and Gertrude van Wagenen, "Compounds Interfering with Ovum Implantation and Development. 3. The role of estrogens," *American Journal of Obstetrics and Gynecology* 96, no. 6 (November 15, 1966): 806–807.
2. Sturgis, quoted in Morris and van Wagenen, "Compounds Interfering with Ovum Implantation," 814.

3. McLennan, quoted in Morris and van Wagenen, "Compounds Interfering with Ovum Implantation," 813.

4. *Griswold v. Connecticut,* 381 U.S. 479 (1965). For more on the evolution of the concept of the right of privacy in American jurisprudence, see David J. Garrow, *Liberty and Sexuality: The Right to Privacy and the Making of Roe v. Wade* (Berkeley: University of California Press, 1998); and John W. Johnson, *Griswold v. Connecticut: Birth Control and the Constitutional Right of Privacy* (Lawrence: University of Kansas Press, 2005).

5. "Family Planning Group Proselytizes," *Yale Daily News,* April 7, 1967, 4–6.

6. Virginia M. Stuermer, "Reflections on Forty Years of Rendering Medical Care to Women," *Yale Journal of Biology and Medicine* 68 (1995): 191–194.

7. Rickie Solinger, *Wake Up Little Susie: Single Pregnancy and Race before Roe v. Wade* (New York and London: Routledge, 1992).

8. Heather Munro Prescott, *"A Doctor of Their Own": The History of Adolescent Medicine* (Cambridge, MA: Harvard University Press, 1998), 149–150.

9. Philip M. Sarrel and Clarence D. Davis, "The Young Unwed Primapara: A Study of 100 Cases with 5 Year Follow-Up," *American Journal of Obstetrics and Gynecology* 95, no. 5 (1966): 722–725; Sarrel, "The University Hospital and the Teenage Unwed Mother," *American Journal of Public Health* 57 (1967): 1312.

10. Leon Speroff, "Bacterial Shock in Obstetrics and Gynecology with Emphasis on Surgical Management of Septic Abortion," *American Journal of Obstetrics and Gynecology* 95, no. 1 (1966): 139–151.

11. Melvin Lewis and Philip M. Sarrel, "Some Psychological Aspects of Seduction, Incest, and Rape in Childhood," *American Academy of Child Psychiatry* 8, no. 4 (1969): 606–619.

12. For more on the history of child sexual abuse, see Hughes Evans, "The Discovery of Child Sexual Abuse in America," in *Formative Years: Children's Health in the United States, 1880–2000,* edited by Alexandra Minna Stern and Howard Markel (Ann Arbor: University of Michigan Press, 2002): 233–259; Evans, "Physician Denial and Child Sexual Abuse in America, 1870–2000," in *Children's Health Issues in Historical Perspective,* edited by Cheryl Krasnick Walsh and Veronica Strong-Boag (Waterloo, Ontario: Wilfrid Laurier Press, 2005): 327–353; and Lynn Sacco, *Unspeakable: Father-Daughter Incest in American History* (Baltimore: Johns Hopkins University Press, 2009). For more on the history of pelvic exams for children and adolescents, see Heather Munro Prescott, "Guides to Womanhood: Gynecology and Adolescent Sexuality in the Post World War II Era," in *Women, Health, and Nation: Canada and the United States since 1945,* edited by Georgina Feldberg, Molly Ladd-Taylor, Alison Li, and Kathryn McPherson (Montreal: McGill-Queen's University Press, 2003), 199–222.

13. Patricia L. N. Donat and John D'Emilio, "A Feminist Redefinition of Rape and Sexual Assault: Historical Foundations and Change," *Journal of Social Issues* 48 (1992): 11–13.

14. Charles R. Hayman, Frances R. Lewis, William F. Stewart, and Murray Grant, "A Public Health Program for Sexually Assaulted Females," *Public Health Reports* 82, no. 6 (1967): 497–504.

15. Harriet F. Pilpel and Nancy F. Wechsler, "Birth Control, Teenagers, and the Law," *Family Planning Perspectives* 1 (1969): 29–36.

16. Quoted in Jane E. Brody, "Human Tests Considered," *New York Times,* May 1, 1966, 1.

17. Joe B. Massey, Celso-Ramon Garcia, and John P. Emich, "Management of Sexually Assaulted Female," *Obstetrics and Gynecology* 38, no. 1 (July 1971): 29–36.

18. Judy Klemesbud, "Yale Students Have Own 'Masters and Johnson,'" *New York Times,* April 28, 1971, 40.

19. Philip M. Sarrel and Lorna J. Sarrel, "A Sex Counseling Service for College Students," *American Journal of Public Health* 61, no. 7 (1971): 1341–1347; Sarrel and Sarrel, "Birth Control Services and Sex Counseling at Yale," *Family Planning Perspectives* 3, no. 3 (July 1971): 33–36. For more on reproductive rights in the Five College region, see David P. Cline, *Creating Choice: A Community Responds to the Need for Abortion and Birth Control, 1961–1973* (New York: Palgrave, 2006).

20. Eleni Skevas and Eric Rosenberg, "DUH's New Gynecology Duo Discuss Sex Counseling Role," *Yale Daily News,* October 16, 1969, 1, 4.

21. "Advice on Sex Offered," *Yale Daily News,* March 4 1970, 1.

22. Shelley Fisher, "Record Number Enrolls in Course on Human Sexuality," *Yale Daily News,* January 29, 1970, 1.

23. Christabelle Sethna, "The Evolution of the Birth Control Handbook: From Student Peer-Education Manual to Feminist Self-Empowerment Text, 1968–1975," *Canadian Bulletin of Medical History/Bulletin canadien d'histoire de la médecine* 23 (2006): 89–117.

24. Eric Rosenberg, "New Sexuality Course Attracts 600 Students," *Yale Daily News,* December 5, 1969, 1–2.

25. Student Committee on Human Sexuality, *Sex and the Yale Student* (New Haven, CT: P. Sarrel, 1970), 15–16, 39–40.

26. Sarrel and Sarrel, "Birth Control Services and Sex Counseling," 33.

27. "Should Colleges Set Up Campus Birth-Control Clinics?" *Glamour,* February 1970, 206.

28. "Contraceptive Counseling, Classes on Sex Seen Needed on Campus," *Ob. Gyn. News,* May 1, 1970, 6.

29. Linda Thurston, *Birth Control, Abortion, and Venereal Disease* (Cambridge, MA: Resist, 1970).

30. Pamela Swift, "Student Sex Clinics," *Philadelphia Sunday Bulletin,* August 29, 1971, clipping from Radcliffe Archives News Office, RG X, Series 7, Box 27, Folder 406, Radcliffe Archives, Schlesinger Library.

31. "Student Guide for Birth Control, Abortion, VD, and Drugs: Resources in the Boston Area," compiled by Larry Berger, Harvard College, 1970, Boston Women's Health Book Collective Papers, Schlesinger Library, Series II, Box 1, Folder 1.13–1.14

32. Copies of these and other manuals can be found in the Takey Crist Papers, Special Collections, Duke University Library, Durham, North Carolina (hereafter referred to as Crist Papers), Box 27. For a review of some of these books, see Takey Crist and Lana Starnes, "Review: Student Printing Presses Bring Birth Control Story to Colleges," *Family Planning Perspectives* 4, no. 1 (1972), 60–61.

33. Henry Woodhead, "At 20, He Teaches 'That Course,'" clipping, *Daily Tar Heel,* ca. 1970, Crist Papers, Box 21.

34. James Trussell and Steve Chandler, *The Loving Book* (Charlotte, NC: Red Clay Pub., 1971). For more on the Institute for the Study of Health and Society, see Naomi Rogers, "'Caution: The AMA May Be Dangerous to Your Health': The Student Health Organizations (SHO) and American Medicine, 1965–1970," *Radical History Review* 80 (2001): 5–34.

35. Carol S., "Important Notice: In Case of Contraceptive Failure, Rape, etc., Get a

Morning-After Contraceptive," *Female Liberation Newsletter,* March 31, 1972, clipping, Women and/in Health Microfilm (Berkeley, CA: Women's History Research Center, ca. 1974, 1975), Section 4, 1763.

36. Thurston, *Birth Control, Abortion, and Venereal Disease,* 8.

37. Lynn K. Hansen, Barbara Reskin, and Diana Gray, *How to Have Intercourse without Getting Screwed* (Seattle, WA: Associated Students of the University of Washington Women's Commission, 1972), 19.

38. Wayne Middendorf and Bruce Middendorf, *A Sperm and Egg Handbook* (Buffalo, NY: SUNY University Press, 1971), 17. Similar advice is given in James L. Burks, MD, and Judith A. Gorbach, *Beyond Eros* (Chicago: University of Chicago Press, 1971), 38–39; Marion Johnson Gray and Roger W. Gray, *How to Take the Worry out of Being Close: An Egg and Sperm Handbook* (Oakland, CA: Son, 1971), 20.

39. Takey Crist, "Contraceptive Practices among College Women," clipping, ca. 1971, Crist Papers, Box 5.

40. Richard Mier, Donald Rollins, Thomas Blush, and Takey Crist, *Elephants and Butterflies . . . and Contraceptives* (Chapel Hill, NC: ECOS, 1970), 11.

41. Quoted in Andrew Malcom, "What They Don't Know about Sex," *New York Times,* August 15, 1971, clipping, Crist papers, Box 5.

42. "The Pill at Stanford," *Time,* November 28, 1969, http://www.time.com/time/magazine/article/0,9171,840431,00.html (accessed June 23, 2010).

43. "The Free-Sex Movement," *Time,* March 11, 1966, 66.

44. "A Morning-After Pill for Absent-Minded Lovers," *San Francisco Chronicle,* October 8, 1969, clipping, Women and/in Health Microfilm (Berkeley, CA: Women's History Research Center, ca. 1974, 1975), 1756.

45. "Birth Control Info at Cowell," *Daily Californian,* September 30, 1965, 2.

46. "Should Colleges Set Up Campus Birth-Control Clinics?" *Glamour,* February 1970, 206.

47. Program Description, PP-WP College Programs, Planned Parenthood Federation of America Papers, Series II, Sophia Smith Collection, Smith College, Northampton, Massachusetts (hereafter referred to as PPFA II Papers), Box 56, Folder 11.

48. For more on the issue of birth control and black allegations of "genocide," see Simone M. Caron, "Birth Control and the Black Community in the 1960s: Genocide or Power Politics?" *Journal of Social History* 31 (1998): 545–559.

49. Gray to Stewart, September 30, 1969, PPFA II Papers, Box 56, Folder 1. For more on Naomi Gray's work, see Jennifer Nelson, *Women of Color and the Reproductive Rights Movement* (New York: New York University Press, 2003), 81–82.

50. Ethel M. Nash, "The Physician's Role in Sex Education," *Journal of the American College Health Association* 15 (May 1967) (Supplement): 69.

51. Quoted in Mary Smith, "Birth Control Pills and the Negro Woman," *Ebony,* March 23, 1968, 34.

52. Woodhead, "At 20, He Teaches 'That Course.'"

53. Donna Cherniak et al., *The Birth Control Handbook,* 4th ed., revised (Montreal: Journal Offset, 1970). For more in the birth control movement in Canadian colleges and universities, see Cristabelle Sethna, "The University of Toronto Health Service, Oral Contraception, and Student Demand for Birth Control, 1960–1970," *Historical Studies in Education* 17 (2005): 265–292; and Sethna, "The Evolution of the *Birth Control Handbook:* From Student Peer Education Manual to Feminist Self-Help Text, 1968–1975," *Canadian Bulletin of Medical History* 23 (1): 89–117.

54. Alan F. Guttmacher and Gene Vadies, "Sex on the Campus and the College Health

Service," paper presented at the Annual Meeting of the American College Health Association, Atlanta, GA, April 6, 1972, PPFA II Papers, Box 56, Folder 15.

55. "Morning After Pill Gets Around," *Medical World News,* December 5, 1969, 13–14.

56. Ibid., 14.

Chapter 3 — Feminist Health Activism and the Feds

1. Lucile Kirtland Kuchera, "Postcoital Contraception with Diethlystilbestrol," *JAMA* 218, no. 4 (25 October 1971): 562.

2. Jane E. Brody, "Success Reported for Next Day Pill," *New York Times,* October 26, 1971, 19.

3. A. L Herbst, H. Ulfelder, and D. C. Poskanzer, "Adenocarcinoma of the Vagina: Association of Maternal Stilbestrol Therapy with Tumor Appearance in Young Women," *New England Journal of Medicine* 284, no. 15 (April 15, 1971): 878–881.

4. Jane Brody, "Disturbing Hints of a Possible Link to Cancer," *New York Times,* October 31, 1971, E14.

5. Morton Mintz, *The Therapeutic Nightmare* (Boston: Beacon Press, 1965); Mintz, *The Pill: An Alarming Report* (Greenwich, CT: Fawcett Publications, 1969). Mintz would later go on to expose corporate malfeasance in the development of the Dalkon Shield intrauterine device in his book *At Any Cost: Corporate Greed, Women, and the Dalkon Shield* (New York: Pantheon Books, 1985).

6. Suzanne White Junod, "Women over 35 Who Smoke: A Case Study in Risk Management and Risk Communication," in *Medicating Modern America: Prescription Drugs in History,* edited by Andrea Tone and Elizabeth Seigel Watkins (New York: New York University Press, 2007), 100–101.

7. Barbara Seaman, *The Doctors' Case against the Pill* (New York: Peter H. Wyden, 1969).

8. Amy Bloom, "The Pill Hearings (1970)," National Women's Health Network website, http://nwhn.org/pill_hearings (accessed June 14, 2010).

9. Elizabeth Watkins, "'Doctor, Are You Trying to Kill Me?' Ambivalence about the Patient Package Insert for Estrogen," *Bulletin of the History of Medicine* 76 (2002): 87–88; Suzanne White Junod and Lara Marks, "Women's Trials: The Approval of the First Contraceptive Pill in the United States and Britain," *Journal of the History of Medicine and Allied Sciences* 57 (2002): 158–159.

10. Alice Echols, *Daring to Be Bad: Radical Feminism in America, 1967–1975* (Minneapolis: University of Minnesota Press, 1989), 93.

11. Kathy Davis, *The Making of Our Bodies, Ourselves: How Feminism Travels across Borders* (Durham, NC: Duke University Press, 2007), 20–21; Sandra Morgen, *Into Our Own Hands: The Women's Health Movement in the United States, 1969–1990* (New Brunswick, NJ: Rutgers University Press, 2002), 16–22; Wendy Kline, *Bodies of Knowledge: Sexuality, Reproduction, and Women's Health in the Second Wave* (Chicago: University of Chicago Press, 2010), 14–16.

12. Quoted in Rita Rubin, "The Pill: 50 Years of Birth Control Changed Women's Lives," *USA Today,* May 9, 2010, http://www.usatoday.com/news/health/2010–05–07–1Api1107_CV_N.htm (accessed August 23, 2010).

13. "'Morning After' Pill Used at U," *Michigan Daily,* undated clipping, Scrapbook, University Health Service Records, Box 4, Bentley History Library, University of Michigan, Ann Arbor, Michigan (hereafter referred to as UHS Records, UMI).

14. Morgen, *Into Our Own Hands,* 10.

15. U.S. Congress, House Subcommittee of the Committee on Government Operations, *Regulation of Diethylstilbestrol (DES) (Its Use as a Drug for Humans and in Animal Feeds),* Part I (Washington, DC: U.S. Government Printing Office, 1972), 52.

16. Transcript of Proceedings, Department of Health, Education, and Welfare, Public Health Service, Food and Drug Administration, Obstetrics and Gynecology Advisory Committee, December 10, 1971, 3–45, FDA History Office, U.S. Food and Drug Administration, Rockville, MD.

17. Kay Weiss, "Cancer and the Morning-After Pill (will you be Mourning-After?)," *her-self* 1 (September 1972): 1.

18. "Fact Sheet: Diethlstilbestrol (DES); The Morning-After Pill," *her-self* 1, no. 7 (1972/73): 14.

19. "Birth Curb Pill Is Termed Risky: Nader Group Reports Coeds Are 'Used as Guinea Pigs," *New York Times,* December 12, 1972, 21. See also "Coeds Said Getting Cancer-Linked Contraceptive," *Durham Morning Herald,* December 12, 1972, clipping, Takey Crist Papers, Special Collections, Duke University Library, Durham, North Carolina (hereafter referred to as Crist Papers), Box 15; "K.U. Clinic Dispenses Morning-After Birth Pill," *Kansas City Times,* December 21, 1972, 6A (courtesy of Jim Swann, FDA History Office); "Ralph Nader Reports: The Morning-After Pill," *Ladies' Home Journal* 90 (1973): 66–67; P. K. "After the Morning After," *Off Our Backs* 34 (December 1972): 8; College Press Service, "Morning After Cancer," *The Great Speckled Bird* 6, no. 10 (March 19, 1973): 10; Kay Weiss, "Afterthoughts on the Morning-After Pill," *Ms.,* November 1973, 22–26.

20. Anita Johnson and Sidney Wolfe to Robben W. Fleming, December 8, 1972, in *Quality of Health Care—Human Experimentation, 1973. Hearings before the Subcommittee on Health of the Committee on Labor and Public Welfare, United States Senate, Ninety-Third Congress* (Washington, DC: U.S. Government Printing Office, 1973), 314–315.

21. Transcript of Proceedings, Department of Health, Education, and Welfare, Public Health Service, Food and Drug Administration, Obstetrics and Gynecology Advisory Committee, January 26, 1973, 34–46.

22. *James H. Jones, Bad Blood: The Tuskegee Syphilis Experiment (New York: Free Press, 1981); Susan M. Reverby, Examining Tuskegee: The Infamous Syphilis Study and Its Legacy (Chapel Hill: University of North Carolina Press, 2009).*

23. Rebecca Kluchin, *Fit to Be Tied: Sterilization and Reproductive Rights in America, 1950–1980* (New Brunswick, NJ: Rutgers University Press, 2009), 155–158.

24. Testimony of Charles Edwards, *Quality of Health Care—Human Experimentation,* 18–49.

25. Testimony of Anita Johnson and Sidney Wolfe, *Quality of Health Care—Human Experimentation,* 193–212.

26. Susan E. Lederer, *Subjected to Science: Human Experimentation in America before the Second World War* (Baltimore: Johns Hopkins University Press, 1995), 139–142.

27. Heather Munro Prescott, "Using Student Bodies: College and University Students as Research Subjects," *Journal of the History of Medicine and Allied Sciences* 57 (2002): 3–38.

28. "Postcoital Diethylstilbestrol," *FDA Drug Bulletin,* May 1973, 1.

29. U.S. House of Representatives, 94th Congress, *Use of Advisory Committees by the Food and Drug Administration* (Washington, DC: Government Printing Office, 1976), 7, 35–40.

30. Belita H. Cowan, "Special Report: The 'Morning-After' Pill," *her-self* 1, no. 4 (September/October 1974): 6–7.

31. Pat Cody, *DES Voices: From Anger to Action* (Columbus: DES Action, 2008), 49–53; Morgen, *Into Our Own Hands,* 30, 156.

32. Fact Sheet on Daughters of DES Mothers, n.d., Boston Women's Health Book Collective Papers, Schlesinger Library, Radcliffe Institute for Advance Study, Cambridge, MA (hereafter referred to as BWHBC Papers), Box 99, FF 9; TO ALL WOMEN BORN BETWEEN 1945–1970: ARE YOU A "D.E.S." DAUGHTER?, BWHBC Papers, Box 100, FF 16.

33. U.S. Senate, *Regulation of Diethylstilbestrol (DES), 1975. Joint Hearing before the Subcommittee on Health of the Committee on Labor and Public Welfare and the Subcommittee on Administrative Practice and Procedure* (Washington, DC: Government Printing Office, 1975), 6–7.

34. Ibid., 14–15.

35. Ibid., 21–26; testimony of Belita H. Cowan on the use of diethylstilbestrol as a 'morning-after' pill, Senate Subcommittee on Health, February 27, 1975, National Women's Health Network Records, Sophia Smith Collection, Smith College, Northampton, MA (hereafter referred to as NWHN Records), Box 7.

36. U.S. Senate, *Regulation of Diethylstilbestrol,* 41–42, 50–51.

37. Ibid., 32–35, 151–160.

38. Ibid., 36–39.

39. Ibid., 26–32. The dispute between officials in the FDA Bureau of Drugs is described in more detail in Diana Dutton, *Worse than the Disease: Pitfalls of Medical Progress* (New York: Cambridge University Press, 1988), 84–85.

40. William A. Nolen, "How Safe Is the 'Morning-After' Pill?," *McCall's* 100 (June 1973): 16, 116.

41. "How Safe Is the Morning-After Birth Control Pill?," *Good Housekeeping* 176 (June 1973): 184.

42. James Dilley to Gene Vadies, January 25, 1973, Planned Parenthood Federation of America Papers, Series II, Sophia Smith Collection, Smith College, Northampton, Massachusetts (hereafter referred to as PPFA II Papers), Box 56, Folder 2.

43. Sandra Grymes, Regional Director, North Atlantic Region, to Mrs. Marcy Lasardi, Executive Director, PP of Northampton County, February 20, 1979, PPFA II Papers, Box 68, Folder 61.

Chapter 4 — Balancing Safety and Choice

1. Philip A. Corfman, "Population Research," *Family Planning Perspectives* 3, no. 4 (1971): 41–42. Corfman describes the origins of the Center for Population Research in "Contraceptives," *Science* n.s. 167 (1970): 1315.

2. Maris A. Vinovskis, *An "Epidemic" of Adolescent Pregnancy? Some Historical and Policy Considerations* (New York: Oxford University Press, 1988).

3. A copy of the RFP (request for proposal) can be found in U.S. Senate Committee on Labor and Public Welfare, Subcommittee on Health, *Quality of Health Care—Human Experimentation, 1973. Hearings before the Subcommittee on Health of the Committee on Labor and Public Welfare, United States Senate, Ninety-third Congress* (Washington, DC: U.S. Government Printing Office, 1973), 135–153.

4. William A. Nolen, "How Safe Is the 'Morning-After' Pill," *McCall's,* June 1973, 16, 116; "How Safe Is the New Morning-After Pill," *Good Housekeeping,* June 1973,

184. Television broadcasts: ABC, September 20, 1973, "FDA/Birth Control Pills"; CBS, September 20, 1973, "FDA/Birth Control Pills"; NBC, September 20, 1973, "FDA/Birth Control Pills"; NBC, February 27, 1975, "Diethylstilbestrol"; CBS, September 9, 1975, "DES Ban." These television news broadcasts are available from the Vanderbilt Media Archives, Vanderbilt University, Nashville, TN. I am very grateful to Suzanne White Junod for telling me about this archive.

5. Mary Henry, "DES Dispute: Contradictory Points of View Swirl over Estrogen's Use as Rape Treatment," *Florida Times-Union,* September 21, 1982, A-1, A-3, National Women's Health Network Records, Sophia Smith Collection, Smith College, Northampton, MA (hereafter referred to as NWHN Records), Box 7.

6. Dianne Glover et al. "Diethylstilbestrol in the Treatment of Rape Victims," *Western Journal of Medicine* 125 (October 1975): 334.

7. "Expert on Cancer Wary of New Pill," *New York Times,* February 23, 1973, 7.

8. Personal communication with Margaret Johnson, November 16, 2010; personal communication with Renee Chelian, January 3, 2011.

9. Kay Weiss, "Afterthoughts on the 'Morning-After' Pill," *Ms.* 2 (November 1973): 26.

10. For more on the radical feminist perspective on rape, see Susan Brownmiller, *In Our Time: Memoir of a Revolution* (New York: Dial Press, 1999), 194–224.

11. Jennifer Nelson, "'All This That Has Happened to Me Shouldn't Happen to Nobody Else': Loretta Ross and the Women of Color Reproductive Freedom Movement of the 1980s," *Journal of Women's History* 22 (2010): 136–160.

12. Maria Bevacqua, "Reconsidering Violence against Women: Coalition Politics in the Antirape Movement," in *Feminist Coalitions: Historical Perspectives on Second-Wave Feminism in the United States,* edited by Stephanie Gilmore (Chicago and Urbana: University of Illinois Press, 2008), 166.

13. Jael Silliman, Marlene Gerber Fried, Loretta Ross, and Elena R. Gutierrez, *Undivided Rights: Women of Color Organize for Reproductive Justice* (Boston: South End Press, 2004).

14. Laura Kaplan, "Beyond Safe and Legal: The Lessons of Jane," in *Abortion Wars: A Half Century of Struggle, 1950–2000,* edited by Rickie Solinger (Berkeley: University of California Press, 1998), 33–41.

15. Richard P. Blye, "The Use of Estrogens as Postcoital Contraceptive Agents," *American Journal of Obstetrics and Gynecology* 116, no. 7 (1973): 1044–1050.

16. Personal communication with Renee Chelian, January 3, 2011.

17. Personal communication with Claire Keyes, November 17, 2010.

18. Minutes, Workshop on Pregnancy Prevention by Estrogens, National Institutes of Health, February 14, 1972, 1, Takey Crist Papers, Special Collections, Duke University Library, Durham, NC, Box 15; Morris and van Wagenen, "Interception: The Use of Postovulatory Estrogens to Prevent Implantation," *American Journal of Obstetrics and Gynecology* 115 (January 1, 1973): 101–106.

19. Minutes, Workshop on Pregnancy Prevention by Estrogens, 2.

20. Ibid.; Takey Crist, "The Use of Estrogen as a Postcoital Contraceptive in North Carolina—Trick or Treatment," *North Carolina Medical Journal* 34, no. 10 (1973): 793–795.

21. Minutes, Workshop on Pregnancy Prevention by Estrogens, 2; Hans Lehfeldt, "Choice of Ethinyl Estradiol as a Postcoital Pill," *American Journal of Obstetrics and Gynecology* 116, no. 6 (July 1973): 892–893; Ary A. Haspels, "The 'Morning-After Pill'—A Preliminary Report," *International Planned Parenthood Federation Bulletin*

3, no. 3 (1969): 6; Haspels, "Post-coital Oestrogen in Large Doses," *International Planned Parenthood Federation* 6, no. 2 (1972): 3–4. Haspels's work with the Amsterdam police comes from Haspels, "Emergency Contraception: A Review," *Contraception* 50 (1994): 101–108.

22. Minutes, Workshop on Pregnancy Prevention by Estrogens, 2–3.

23. Transcript of Proceedings, Department of Health, Education, and Welfare, Public Health Service, Food and Drug Administration, Obstetrics and Gynecology Advisory Committee, March 17, 1972, 18–43.

24. Garrett Dixon, James J. Schlesselman, Howard W. Ory, and Richard P. Blye, "Ethinyl Estradiol and Conjugated Estrogens as Postcoital Contraceptives," *JAMA* 244, no. 12 (September 19, 1980): 1336–1337.

25. Ibid., 1337–1338.

26. Ibid., 1338–1339.

27. Morris Notelovitz and David Sayre Bard, "Conjugated Estrogen as Post-ovulatory Interceptive," *Contraception* 17, no. 5 (May 1978): 443–454.

28. "Beginnings," *Network News,* October 1976, 1, NWHN Records, Box 6.

29. Wendy Kline, *Bodies of Knowledge: Sexuality, Reproduction, and Women's Health in the Second Wave* (Chicago: University of Chicago Press, 2010), 4–5.

30. Testimony of Judy Norsigian presented on behalf of the National Women's Health Network, Hearings before the House Select Committee on Population March 8, 1978, in U.S. Congress, House Select Committee on Population, *Fertility and Contraception in America: Contraceptive Technology and Development*, vol. 3 (Washington, DC: Government Printing Office, 1978), 375–379.

31. Ibid.

32. Ibid.

33. Minutes of Fertility and Maternal Health Drugs Advisory Committee, Food and Drug Administration, April 11, 1980, 42–43, NWHN Records, Box 7.

34. Barbara Resnick Troetel, "Three-Part Disharmony: The Transformation of the Food and Drug Administration in the 1970s" (PhD diss., City University of New York, 1996).

35. Personal communication with Claire Keyes, November 17, 2010. For more on the history of menstrual extraction, see Rebecca Chalker and Carol Downer, *A Woman's Book of Choices: Abortion, RU-486, Menstrual Extraction* (Village Station, NY: Four Walls Eight Windows, 1992), 113–128.

36. Minutes of Fertility and Maternal Health Drugs Advisory Committee, Food and Drug Administration, April 11, 1980, 26–33.

37. Ibid., 34–37.

38. Ibid., 55–57.

39. Ibid., 44–45.

40. Ibid., 91–92.

41. "Postcoital Estrogens Win Backing of FDA Advisers," *Medical World News* 21, no. 11 (May 26, 1980): 26.

42. Cristabelle Sethna, "The Evolution of the 'Birth Control Handbook': From Student Peer-Education Manual to Feminist Self-Empowerment Text, 1968–1975," *Canadian Bulletin of the History of Medicine* 23, no. 1 (2006): 89–117; Sethna, "The University of Toronto Health Service, Oral Contraception, and Student Demand for Birth Control, 1960–1970," *Historical Studies in Education* 17, no. 2 (2005): 265–292.

43. Angus McLaren and Arlene Tigar McLaren, *The Bedroom and the State: The Changing Practices and Politics of Contraception and Abortion in Canada, 1880–1997* (Toronto and New York: Oxford University Press, 1997).

44. Author interview with A. Albert Yuzpe, September 24, 2009.
45. A. A. Yuzpe et al., "Post Coital Contraception—A Pilot Study," *Journal of Reproductive Medicine* 13, no. 2 (1974): 53–58; Yuzpe and William J. Lancee, "Ethinylestradiol and dl-Norgestral as a Postcoital Contraceptive," *Fertility and Sterility* 28, no. 9 (September 1977): 932–936; Yuzpe, "Postcoital Hormonal Contraception: Uses, Risks, Abuses," *International Journal of Gynaecology and Obstetrics* 15, no. 2 (1977): 133–136; R. Percival Smith and Adrianne Ross, "Post-coital Contraception Using Dl-Norgestral/Ethinyl Estradiol Combination," *Contraception* 17, no. 3 (1978): 247–252.
46. Lee H. Schilling, "An Alternative to the Use of High-Dose Estrogens of Postcoital Contraception," *Journal of the American College Health Association* 27 (1979): 247–249. See also Schilling, "Awareness of the Existence of Postcoital Contraception among Students Who Have Had a Therapeutic Abortion," *Journal of American College Health* 32 (1984): 244–246.
47. "Ovral Touted as Morning-After Pill," *Contraceptive Technology Update* 1, no. 1 (April 1980): 11–13.
48. James Trussell and Robert A. Hatcher, *Women in Need* (New York: Macmillan, 1972), 148–151.
49. Karen Poirier-Brode, "In Memorium: Felicia Hance Stewart," *Sierra Sacramento Valley Medicine* 57, no. 4 (2006), http://www.ssvms.org/ssv_medicine/archives/2006/04/articles/0604-obit-stewart.pdf (accessed August 19, 2010); Felicia Hance Stewart, *My Body, My Health: The Concerned Woman's Book of Gynecology* (Sacramento, CA: Consumer Union, 1979).
50. Robert A. Hatcher, "Morning-After Pill Can Unlock Health Care Door," *Contraceptive Technology Update* 1, no. 4 (July 1980): 54.
51. Author interview with A. Albert Yuzpe, September 24, 2009.
52. "Postcoital Contraception: A Delicate Political Issue," *Contraceptive Technology Update* 5, no. 4 (April 1984): 41–43.
53. "Lack of Data on 'Morning After' Pill Confounds Clinicians," *Contraceptive Technology Update* 8, no. 11 (November 1987): 137–139.
54. "Lack of Awareness Reason Most Do Not Prescribe Postcoital OCs," *Contraceptive Technology Update* 7, no. 9 (September 1986): 106–107.
55. Eve W. Paul, director of Legal Services, to Mr. Jack Shettle, Brooks, Shettle & Garman, September 20, 1978; Eve W. Paul to Winston Gaye, July 27, 1978, Planned Parenthood Federation of America Papers, Series II, Sophia Smith Collection, Smith College, Northampton, MA, Box 68, Folder 61.
56. Personal communication with Claire Keyes, December 10, 2010; personal communication with Renee Chelian, January 3, 2011.

Chapter 5 — Building Consensus

1. Belita Cowan, "Ethical Problems in Government-Funded Research," in *Birth Control and Controlling Birth*, edited by Helen B. Holmes, Betty B. Hoskins, and Michael Gross (Clifton, NJ: Human Press, 1980), 37–46.
2. Helen Holmes, "Reproductive Technologies: The Birth of a Women-Center Analysis," in *Birth Control and Controlling Birth*, edited by Holmes, Hoskins, and Gross, 16.
3. Ibid.
4. Kristen Luker, reply to "Ethical Problems in Government-Funded Research," in *Birth Control and Controlling Birth*, edited by Holmes, Hoskins, and Gross, 81–83.
5. *Roe v. Wade*, 410 U.S. 113 (1973).

6. *Harris v. McRae,* 448 U.S. 297 (1980); *Bowen v. Kendrick,* 487 U.S. 589 (1988); *Webster v. Reproductive Health Services,* 492 U.S. 490 (1989); Rickie Solinger, ed., *Abortion Wars: A Half Century of Struggle, 1950–2000* (Berkeley: University of California Press, 1998), xiii–xiv.

7. Historical background comes from "NARAL's New Way: Women in Politics," *Southern Exposure* 12, no. 1 (1984): 26–31.

8. Jennifer Nelson, *Women of Color and the Reproductive Rights Movement* (New York: New York University Press, 2003), 133–177.

9. Marie Bass, "Toward Coalition: The Reproductive Health Technologies Project," in *Abortion Wars,* edited by Solinger, 252–254.

10. David A. Grimes et al., "Early Abortion with a Single Dose of the Antiprogestin RU 486," *American Journal of Obstetrics and Gynecology* 158 (1988): 1307–1312.

11. Bass, "Toward Coalition," 254.

12. Sarah Weddington to Marie Bass, October 20, 1987, Bass and Howes Papers, Acc# 2004-M56, Schlesinger Library, Radcliffe Institute for Advanced Study, Cambridge, MA (hereafter referred to as Bass and Howes Papers), Box 11.

13. "Proposed Plan of Action," 1989, 2. Bass and Howes Papers, Box 34a.

14. Marie Bass, Joanne Howes, and Nanette Falkenberg, *A Report on RU 486 and Its Prospects for Use in the United States* (Washington, DC: Bass and Howes, 1987).

15. Joanne Howes to Al Moran, May 23, 1988, Bass and Howes Papers, Box 11.

16. "Proposed Plan of Action," 4.

17. Bass, "Toward Coalition," 258–259.

18. Ibid., 257.

19. Transcript of interview of Sharon Camp by Rebecca Sharpless, August 20–21, 2003, Population and Reproductive Health Oral History Project, Sophia Smith Collection, Smith College (hereafter referred to as Camp interview), 25.

20. "Marie's Speech," 1991, Bass and Howes Papers, Box 34a.

21. Transcript of interview of Loretta Ross by Joyce Follett, November 3–5, 2004, December 1–3, 2004, Voices of Feminism Project, Sophia Smith Collection, Smith College, 76–78.

22. Loretta Ross, "RU-486: Are You Sure or RU Sure You Want It?," draft manuscript, n.d., Loretta Ross Papers, Sophia Smith Collection, Smith College, Box 2.

23. Bass, "Toward Coalition," 359–361.

24. Ibid., 359–361.

25. "Proposed Plan of Action," 8.

26. Marie Bass to Malcolm Potts, President, Family Health International, March 1, 1989, Bass and Howes Papers, Box 11a.

27. Bass, "Toward Coalition," 262–264.

28. Board Biographies, Bass and Howes Papers, Box 11a.

29. Bass, "Toward Coalition," 262–264.

30. *American Agenda,* "Medicine: The Morning-After Pill," ABC World News, January 5, 1994, Vanderbilt Television News Archive, Nashville, TN.

31. Personal communication with Marie Bass, September 27, 2010.

32. Minutes of Board Meeting, March 5, 1993, Bass and Howes Papers, Box 40.

33. Quoted in "Women Already Have a Choice, They Just Don't Know It," Press Release, 1994. Bass and Howes Papers, Box 11a.

34. Progress Report, Task Force on Postcoital Contraception, March 4, 1994, Bass and Howes Papers, Box 40a.

35. Minutes of Board Meeting, March 5, 1993.

36. Jan Hoffman, "The Morning After Pill: A Well Kept Secret," *New York Times*, January 10, 1993, Sec. 6, p. 12; Peter Jaret, "The Morning-After Pill," *Glamour*, September 1992, 61; Marie McCullough, "Morning-After Pill Exists, Yet Few Women Know It," *Philadelphia Inquirer*, June 1, 1994, A1; Carol Ostrom, "A Little Contraception Pill That's a Big Unknown," *Seattle Times*, July 2, 1993, A1.

37. Lisa L. Wynn, "US: Sexual Archetypes from the DIY to Post-Dedicated Product Eras," in *Emergency Contraception: The Story of a Global Reproductive Health Technology*, edited by Angel M. Foster and L. L. Wynn (New York: Palgrave Macmillan, forthcoming).

38. Personal communication with Renee Chelian, January 3, 2011.

39. Memorandum to Affiliate Executive Directors and Affiliate Medical Directors from Louise B. Tyrer and Julie E. Salas, January 13, 1988, Felicia Hance Stewart Papers, Acc#2006-M109, Schlesinger Library, Radcliffe Institute for Advanced Study, Cambridge, MA, Box 1.

40. Alison Piepmeier, *Girl Zines: Making Media, Doing Feminism* (New York: New York University Press, 2009), 191.

41. Robert Hatcher, A. J. Trussell, F. Stewart, et. al. *Emergency Contraception: The Nation's Best-Kept Secret* (Decataur, GA: Bridging the Gap Communications, 1995).

42. James Trussell, Jessica Bull, Jacqueline Koenig, Marie Bass, Amy Allina, and Vanessa Northington Gamble, "Call 1–888-NOT-2-LATE: Promoting Emergency Contraception in the United States," *Journal of the American Medical Women's Association* 53, no. 5, Supplement 2 (1998): 247–250; Francine Coeytaux and Barbara Pillsbury, "Bringing Emergency Contraception to American Women: The History and Remaining Challenges," *Women's Health Issues* 11, no. 2 (2001): 82.

43. James Trussell, Felicia Stewart, Felicia Guest, and Robert A. Hatcher, "Emergency Contraceptive Pills: A Simple Proposal to Reduce Unintended Pregnancies," *Family Planning Perspectives* 24 (1992): 269–273.

44. Joyce Price, "Report Says Several Drugs Can Act as Abortion Pills," *Washington Times*, January 3, 1993, A5.

45. Judy Norsigian, "Her Say: Don't Make the Pill Easier to Acquire," *Chicago Tribune*, April 11, 1993, Section 8, 9.

46. Elyse Tanouye and Rose Gutfeld, "Health: Talks Cancelled on Making 'Pill' Nonprescription," *Wall Street Journal*, January 28, 1993, B1.

47. Norsigian, "Her Say: Don't Make the Pill Easier to Acquire," Section 8, 9.

48. For more on the history of efforts to make oral contraceptives available over the counter, see Heather Munro Prescott, "Safer Than Aspirin: The Campaign for Over-the-Counter Oral Contraceptives," in *The Prescription in Perspective: Therapeutic Authority in Late 20th Century America*, edited by Jeremy A. Greene and Elizabeth Siegel Watkins (Baltimore: Johns Hopkins University Press, forthcoming).

49. Board Biographies, Bass and Howes Papers, Box 11a.

50. National Women's Health Network, "Position Paper: Postcoital Contraception: Time for Cautious Approval," 1993,National Women's Health Network Records, Sophia Smith Collection, Smith College, Northampton, MA, Box 7. For more on the network's continuing opposition to OTC status for oral contraceptives, see "Network's Position on Oral Contraceptive Availability without a Prescription," *Network News*, May/June 1993, 5, 7–8.

51. Camp interview, 64.

Chapter 6 — Mainstreaming Emergency Contraception

1. *ER,* "Tribes" (broadcast April 10, 1997), Internet Movie Database.
2. Henry J. Kaiser Family Foundation, *National Survey Results on Public Knowledge/ Opinions and OB/GYN Practice/Attitudes on Emergency Contraceptives ("Morning-After Pills"),* publication number 1044, publish date, March 3, 1995, http://www. kff.org/womenshealth/1044-index.cfm (accessed May 28, 2010).
3. Susan Ferraro, "Right About Now You Might be Interested in Learning About Emergency Contraception," *New York Daily News,* August 21, 1997, 59.
4. Henry J. Kaiser Family Foundation, *Documenting the Power of Television—A Survey of Regular E.R. Viewers about Emergency Contraception,* publication number 1358, publish date, June 1, 1997, http://www.kff.org/womenshealth/1358-index.cfm (accessed May 28, 2010).
5. L. L. Wynn, "US: Sexual Archetypes from the DIY to Post-Dedicated Product Eras," in *Emergency Contraception: The Story of a Global Reproductive Health Technology,* edited by Angel M. Foster and L. L. Wynn (New York: Palgrave Macmillan, 2010).
6. Barbara Pillsbury, Francine Coeytaux, and Andrea Johnson, *From Secret to Shelf: How Collaboration Is Bringing Emergency Contraception to Women* (Los Angeles: Pacific Institute for Women's Health, 1999), 12.
7. Cited in Francine Coeytaux and Barbara Pillsbury, "Bringing Emergency Contraception to American Women: The History and Remaining Challenges," *Women's Health Issues* 11, no. 2 (2001): 82.
8. "First Emergency Contraceptive Product Hits U.S. Market Shelves," *Contraceptive Technology Update* 19, no. 11 (1998): 141.
9. Transcript of interview of Sharon Camp by Rebecca Sharpless, August 20–21, 2003, Population and Reproductive Health Oral History Project, Sophia Smith Collection, Smith College (hereafter referred to as Camp interview), 71.
10. Quoted in Philip J. Hilts, "Birth-Control Backlash," *New York Times,* December 16, 1990, SM41.
11. "Roderick L. Mackenzie on the Development of Gynetics and the Emergency Contraceptive Kit," Business News New Jersey, September 21, 1998, http://findarticles. com/p/articles/mi_qa6206/is_199809/ai_n24343442/?tag=content;c011 (accessed June 23, 2010).
12. Marie Bass to Roderick L. Mackenzie, March 7, 1989, Bass and Howes Papers, Acc# 2004-M56, Schlesinger Library, Radcliffe Institute for Advanced Study, Cambridge, MA, Box 11a.
13. United States, Congress, House, Committee on Small Business, Subcommitte on Regulation, Business Opportunitites, and Energy, *The Safety and Effectiveness of the Abortifacient RU486 in Foreign Markets: Opportunities and Obstacles to U.S. Commercialization: Hearing before the Subcommittee on Regulation, Business Opportunities, and Energy of the Committee on Small Business, House of Representatives, One Hundred Second Congress, First Session, Washington, DC, December 5, 1991* (Washington, DC: Government Printing Office, 1991), 308.
14. Agnes Donahue to Dr. Mason, March 5, 1991, Office of Women's Health Records, Acc# 2001–077, National Library of Medicine, Bethesda, MD, Box 2, Folder 1.
15. Marie Bass and Joanne Howes, "Women's Health: The Making of a Powerful New Public Issue," *Women's Health Issues* 2 (1992): 3–5.
16. Joanne Howes and Marie Bass, "A Significant Day for Women's Health and the FDA," *Journal of Gender Specific Medicine* 1 (1998): 14–15, 17.
17. Janet Benshoof, Simon Heller, and Diane Curtis, "Citizen's Petition, Memorandum

of Law in the Matter of Misbranded Oral Contraceptives," November 23, 1994, 1, Docket 94P-0427/CP 1, FDA Dockets Management Branch.

18. Arthur A. Daemmrich, *Pharmacopolitics: Drug Regulation in the United States and Germany* (Chapel Hill: University of North Carolina, 2004), 30–32.

19. Benshoof, Heller, and Curtis, "Citizen's Petition, Memorandum of Law," 2.

20. Ibid., 9–11.

21. Ibid., 11.

22. Barbara A. Nevergold and Colleen Brown, Planned Parenthood of Buffalo and Erie County, to David Kessler, May 17, 1995, Docket 94P-0427/CP 1, FDA Dockets Management Branch.

23. Deposition of David Grimes, In the Matter of Misbranded Oral Contraceptives, Docket 94P-0427/CP 1, FDA Dockets Management Branch.

24. Deposition of Jane E. Hodgson, Docket 94P-0427/CP 1, FDA Dockets Management Branch.

25. Janet Woodcock to Benshoof, Heller, and Curtis, March 9, 1996, Docket 94P-0427/CP 1, FDA Dockets Management Branch.

26. Reproductive Health Drugs Advisory Committee Minutes, June 28, 1996, FDA Center for Drug Evaluation and Research.

27. Quoted in Marie McCullough, "Pill Use Backed for After-Sex Birth Control," *Philadelphia Inquirer,* February 25, 1997, A01.

28. Quoted in Tamar Lewin, "Agency Wants the Pill Redefined," *New York Times,* July 1, 1996, A1, B6.

29. David A. Kessler, "Prescription Drug Products: Certain Combined Oral Contraceptives for Use as Postcoital Emergency Contraceptives," *Federal Register* 62, no. 37 (1997): 8610–8612.

30. Quoted in John Schwartz, "FDA Backs New Use for the Pill; 'Morning-After' Doses Get 1st Endorsement," *Washington Post,* February 25, 1997, A01.

31. Quoted in Peter Keeting, "Where Drug Companies Fear to Tread: The Long, Strange Journey of Preven," *Fortune* 138, no. 8 (October 26, 1998), 48.

32. McCullough, "Pill Use Backed for After-Sex Birth Control," A01.

33. Quoted in Keeting, "Where Drug Companies Fear to Tread," 48.

34. Quoted in McCullough, "Pill Use Backed for After-Sex Birth Control," A01.

35. Quoted in Keeting, "Where Drug Companies Fear to Tread."

36. Quoted in "First Emergency Contraceptive Product Hits U.S. Market Shelves," *Contraceptive Technology Update* 19, 1no. 1 (1998): 141–143.

37. Ilina Singh, "Not Just Naughty: 50 Years of Stimulant Drug Advertising," in *Medicating Modern America: Prescription Drugs in History,* edited by Andrea Tone and Elizabeth Siegel Watkins (New York: New York University Press, 2007), 148–149.

38. "Morning After," Advertising Age 69, no. 43 (October 26, 1998), 52.

39. "Companies Commit to Emergency Contraception—Have You? "*Contraceptive Technology Update* 20, no. 12 (1999): 137.

40. Quoted in Press Release, GYNÉTICS INC. LAUNCHES CONSUMER MARKETING CAMPAIGN TO SUPPORT PREVEN™ EMERGENCY CONTRACEPTIVE KIT, October 28, 1998, http://web.archive.org/web/19990504201502/www.preven.com/press/04-02b.html (accessed June 7, 2010).

41. Feminist Daily Newswire, March 17, 1999, http://www.feminist.org/news/newsbyte/uswirestory.asp?id=2186 (accessed March 24, 2005).

42. Quoted in Elyse Tanouye, "FDA Approves Kit to Prevent Pregnancies," *Wall Street Journal,* September 3, 1998, B1.

43. Quoted in Susan Ferraro, "Sex and the Single Pill: Morning-After Contraception Is About to Become Easier and More Effective," *New York Daily News*, August 20, 1998, 60.

44. P. C. and M.S.W. Kwan, "A Prospective Randomized Comparison of Levonorgestral and the Yuzpe Regimen in Post-Coital Contraception," *Human Reproduction* 8 (1993): 389–392.

45. Author's interview with Sharon Camp, March 17, 2005.

46. ISEC website, http://www.cecinfo.org/.

47. Camp interview, 69, 72.

48. Ibid., 77–78.

49. Ibid., 78–80.

50. Wynn, "US: Sexual Archetypes from the DIY to Post-Dedicated Product Eras."

51. "About the Consortium," Felicia Hance Stewart Papers, Acc#2006-M109, Schlesinger Library, Radcliffe Institute for Advanced Study, Cambridge, MA, Box 1; Emergency Contraception Update, March 1998, http://www.cecinfo.org/publications/newsletter.htm (accessed November 12, 2010).

52. Camp interview, 83–84.

53. Quoted in "Emergency Contraception Use Up—New ECP Arrives," *Contraceptive Technology Update* 20, no. 9 (September 1999): 108.

54. Sarah J. Heim, "DDB Pushes Morning-After Pill: With Limited Funds, Plan B Marketer Focuses on College Women," *ADWEEK Western Edition* 52 (February 11, 2002): 5.

Chapter 7 — From Paternalism to Patient Empowerment

1. Quoted in Barbara Pillsbury, Francine Coeytaux, and Andrea Johnson, *From Secret to Shelf: How Collaboration Is Bringing Emergency Contraception to Women* (Los Angeles: Pacific Institute for Women's Health, 1999), 29.

2. Davina C. Ling, Ernst R. Berndt and Margaret K. Kyle, "Deregulating Direct-to-Consumer Marketing of Prescription Drugs: Effects on Prescription and Over-the-Counter Product Sales," *Journal of Law and Economics* 45 (2002): 691–692.

3. R. William Soller, "Evolution of Self-Care with Over-the-Counter Medications," *Clinical Therapeutics* 20 (1998): Supplement C, C134–140.

4. Geoffrey Cowle, "Right Off the Shelf," *Newsweek,* July 10, 2000, 50.

5. James Trussell, Felicia Stewart, Felicia Guest, Robert A. Hatcher, "Emergency Contraceptive Pills: A Simple Proposal to Reduce Unintended Pregnancies," *Family Planning Perspectives* 24 (1992): 269–273.

6. James Trussell, Felicia Stewart, Felicia Guest, Charlotte Ellertson, and Malcolm Potts, "Efficacy Implications of Making the Pill Available Over the Counter," in *The Pill from Prescription to Over the Counter* (Menlo Park, CA: Henry J. Kaiser Foundation, 1994), 121, 130.

7. Quoted in Michael McMahon, "Pondering a Non-prescription Pill," *USA Today,* March 16, 1992, 4D.

8. For more on the history of efforts to make oral contraceptives available over the counter, see Heather Munro Prescott, "Safer Than Aspirin: The Campaign for Over-the-Counter Oral Contraceptives," in *The Prescription in Perspective: Therapeutic Authority in Late 20th Century America,* edited by Jeremy A. Greene and Elizabeth Siegel Watkins (Baltimore: Johns Hopkins University Press, forthcoming).

9. Elisa S. Wells, Jane Hutchings, Jacqueline S. Gardner, Jennifer L. Winkler, Timothy

S. Fuller, Don Downing, and Rod Shafer, "Using Pharmacies in Washington State to Expand Access to Emergency Contraception," *Family Planning Perspectives* 30 (1998): 288–290.

10. Gina Kolata, "Without Fanfare, Morning-After Pill Gets a Closer Look," *New York Times,* October 8, 2000, 1, 22.

11. Quoted in Dana Canedy, "Wal-Mart Decides against Selling a Contraceptive," *New York Times,* May 14, 1999, C1.

12. "Over-the-Counter Drug Products; Public Hearing," *Federal Register* 65, no. 82 (April 27, 2000): 24704–24706.

13. Sarah Lueck, "FDA Examines More Switches of Drugs to Be Nonprescription," Wall Street Journal (Eastern edition), June 29, 2000, B26.

14. Kirsten Moore, Comments before Food and Drug Administration Public Hearing on Over-the-Counter Drug Products, June 28, 2000, Docket 00N-1256, www.fda.gov/ohrms/dockets/DOCKETS/00n1256/ts00013.pdf (accessed June 22, 2010).

15. Tara Shocket, Comments before Food and Drug Administration Public Hearing on Over-the-Counter Drug Products, June 28, 2000, Docket 00N-1256, www.fda.gov/ohrms/dockets/DOCKETS/00n1256/ts00013.pdf (accessed June 22, 2010).

16. Jack Stover, Comments before Food and Drug Administration Public Hearing on Over-the-Counter Drug Products, June 28, 2000, Docket 00N-1256, www.fda.gov/ohrms/dockets/DOCKETS/00n1256/ts00013.pdf (accessed June 22, 2010).

17. Amy Allina, Comments before Food and Drug Administration Public Hearing on Over-the-Counter Drug Products, June 28, 2000, Docket 00N-1256, www.fda.gov/ohrms/dockets/DOCKETS/00n1256/ts00013.pdf (accessed June 22, 2010).

18. Ibid.

19. Ibid.

20. Susan Lavine Coleman, Comments before Food and Drug Administration Public Hearing on Over-the-Counter Drug Products, June 28, 2000, Docket 00N-1256, www.fda.gov/ohrms/dockets/DOCKETS/00n1256/ts00013.pdf (accessed June 22, 2010).

21. Quoted in Rita Rubin, "Emergency Contraception Remains Rare Prescriptions, Doctors' Silence Limit Pills' Use," *USA Today,* November 15, 2000, 11D.

22. Citizens Petition, February 14, 2001, Docket FDA-2001-P-0123 (all FDA dockets are available at www.regulations.gov).

23. Affidavit by David Grimes and Raymond, Docket FDA-2001-P-0123.

24. Letter from Randall W. Lutter to Bonnie Scott Jones and Simon Heller, June 9, 2006, Docket No. 2001P-0075/CP1.

25. Lisa L. Wynn, "US: Sexual Archetypes from the DIY to Post-dedicated Product Eras," in *Emergency Contraception: The Story of a Global Reproductive Health Technology,* edited by Angel M. Foster and L. L. Wynn (New York: Palgrave Macmillan, forthcoming).

26. Transcript of United States of America Food and Drug Administration Center for Drug Evaluation and Research Nonprescription Drugs Advisory Committee (NDAC) in Joint Session with the Advisory Committee for Reproductive Health Drugs (ACRHD), December 16, 2003, http://www.fda.gov/ohrms/dockets/ac/03/transcripts/4015T1.htm (accessed June 22, 2010).

27. Ibid.

28. Wynn, "US: Sexual Archetypes."

29. Transcript of United States of America Food and Drug Administration Center for Drug Evaluation and Research Nonprescription Drugs Advisory Committee (NDAC) in Joint Session with the Advisory Committee for Reproductive Health

Drugs (ACRHD), December 16, 2003, http://www.fda.gov/ohrms/dockets/ac/03/transcripts/4015T1.htm (accessed June 22, 2010).

30. Quoted in "FDA Advisory Panels Recommend EC Be Sold without Prescription," *Kaiser Daily Women's Health Policy,* December 17, 2003, http://www.kaisernetwork.org/daily_reports/rep_index.cfm?DR_ID=21382 (accessed June 22, 2010).

31. Letter from Randall W. Lutter to Bonnie Scott Jones and Simon Heller, June 9, 2006, Docket No. 2001P-0075/CP1.

32. Quoted in L. L. Wynn, Joanna N. Erdman, Angel M. Foster, and James Trussell, "Harm Reduction or Women's Rights? Debating Access to Emergency Contraceptive Pills in Canada and the United States," *Studies in Family Planning* 38 (2007): 254.

33. Quoted in Wynn et al., "Harm Reduction or Women's Rights?" 254.

34. Center for Reproductive Rights, "Center for Reproductive Rights Questions Timing of Plan B Announcement," July 31, 2006, http://reproductiverights.org/en/pressroom/center-for-reproductive-rights-questions-timing-of-fda-plan-b-announcement (accessed June 22, 2010).

35. "Morning-After Pill Conspiracy: Interview with Annie Tummino," http://reproductiverights.org/en/document/morning-after-pill-conspiracy-interview-with-annie-tummino (accessed June 22, 2010).

36. Morning-After Pill Conspiracy—History, http://www.mapconspiracy.org/history.html (accessed June 22, 2010).

37. Jenny Brown, "One Million March for Women s Reproductive Rights," May 15, 2004, http://jfbrown.wordpress.com/2004/05/15/one-million-march-for-womens-reproductive-rights/ (accessed June 23, 2010).

38. Morning-After Pill Conspiracy to Steven Galison, June 10, 2004, http://www.fda.gov/ohrms/dockets/dailys/04/aug04/082604/01p-0075-c002022–01-v01289.pdf (accessed October 29, 2010).

39. Morning-After Pill Conspiracy—History.

40. "Morning-After Pill Conspiracy: Interview with Annie Tummino."

41. Morning-After Pill Conspiracy—History.

42. Jenny Brown, "FDA Tries to Divide Women by Age to Deny Us Our Rights!," http://www.mapconspiracy.org/age.html (accessed June 22, 2010).

43. Quoted in Gardner Harris, "Official Quits on Pill Delay at the F.D.A.," *New York Times,* September 1, 2005, A12.

44. United States Government Accountability Office, *Decision Process to Deny Initial Application for Over-the-Counter Marketing of the Emergency Contraceptive Drug Plan B Was Unusual,* GAO-06–109, November 14, 2005, http://www.gao.gov/new.items/d06109.pdf (accessed June 22, 2010).

45. Quoted in "Former Head of FDA to be Deposed on Tuesday in 'Morning-After Pill' Case as Agency Rejects Five-Year-Old Citizen's Petition," http://reproductiverights.org/en/press-room/former-head-of-fda-to-be-deposed-on-tuesday-in-morning-after-pill-case-as-agency-rejects (accessed June 23, 2010).

46. See http://reproductiverights.org/en/document/federal-court-rules-fda-must-reconsider-plan-b-decision-0.

47. See http://www.mapconspiracy.org/ (accessed June 23, 2010).

48. Quoted in "FDA Approves Plan B for 17 year olds," *Contemporary Sexuality* 43, no. 6 (2009): 12.

49. Center for Reproductive Rights, Memorandum of Law in Support of Plaintiff's Motion for Civil Contempt, November 16, 2010, http://reproductiverights.org/sites/

crr.civicactions.net/files/documents/Mem%20in%20Support%200f%20Motion%2
0for%20Contempt%20FINAL%2011–16–10%20830am.pdf (accessed November 22,
2010).

50. Amy Allina, "Sex and Science at the Food and Drug Administration," *Women's
Health Activist* 35, no. 6 (2010): 1, 3.

Conclusion

1. Francine Coeytaux, Elisa S. Wells, and Elizabeth Westley, "Editorial: Emergency
Contraception: Have We Come Full Circle?" *Contraception* 80 (2009): 1–3.
2. Sandra Levy," The New Gatekeepers: Changing Market Conditions Are Catapulting
Pharmacists into the Pivotal Role of Patrolling a Third Class of Drugs," *Drug Topics*
25 (July 2005): 24.
3. Transcript of United States of America Food and Drug Administration Center
for Drug Evaluation and Research Nonprescription Drugs Advisory Committee
(NDAC) in Joint Session with the Advisory Committee for Reproductive Health
Drugs (ACRHD), December 16, 2003, http://www.fda.gov/ohrms/dockets/ac/03/
transcripts/4015T1.htm (accessed June 22, 2010).
4. Wendy Kline, *Bodies of Knowledge: Sexuality, Reproduction, and Women's Health
in the Second Wave* (Chicago: University of Chicago Press, 2010); Susan Reverby,
"Thinking through the Body and the Body Politic: Feminism, History, and Health-
Care Policy in the United States," in *Women, Health, and Nation: Canada and the
United States since 1945,* edited by Georgina Feldberg, Molly Ladd-Taylor, Alison
Li, and Kathryn McPherson (Montreal: McGill-Queen's University Press, 2003),
404–420.
5. Working group participants include representatives from the National Women's
Health Network and other former critics of the OTC switch. Statement of Purpose,
Oral Contraceptives Over-the-Counter Working Group, http://ocsotc.org/?page_id=5
(accessed July 13, 2010).
6. Behind the Counter Availability of Certain Drugs, Public Meeting, Wednesday,
November 14, 2007, Transcript, Docket FDA-2007-N-00832, www.regulations.gov.

Index

Available titles in the Critical Issues in Health and Medicine series: